THE INTERNATIONAL SERIES OF MONOGRAPHS ON CHEMISTRY

1. J.D. Lambert: *Vibrational and rotational relaxation in gases*
2. N.G. Parsonage and L.A.K. Staveley: *Disorder in crystals*
3. G.C. Maitland, M. Rigby, E.B. Smith, and W.A. Wakeham: *Intermolecular forces: their origin and determination*
4. W.G. Richards, H.P. Trivedi, and D.L. Cooper: *Spin–orbit coupling in molecules*
5. C.F. Cullis and M.M. Hirschler: *The combustion of organic polymers*
6. R.T. Bailey, A.M. North, and R.A. Pethrick: *Molecular motion in high polymers*
7. Atta-ur-Rahman and A. Basha: *Biosynthesis of indole alkaloids*
8. J.S. Rowlinson and B. Widom: *Molecular theory of capillarity*
9. C.G. Gray and K.E. Gubbins: *Theory of molecular fluids. Volume 1: Fundamentals*
10. C.G. Gray and K.E. Gubbins: *Theory of molecular fluids. Volume 2: Applications*
11. S. Wilson: *Electron correlation of molecules*
12. E. Haslam: *Metabolites and metabolism*

Metabolites and Metabolism

A commentary on secondary metabolism

Edwin Haslam

*Department of Chemistry,
University of Sheffield*

Clarendon Press · Oxford
1985

Oxford University Press, Walton Street, Oxford OX2 6DP

London New York Toronto
Delhi Bombay Calcutta Madras Karachi
Kuala Lumpur Singapore Hong Kong Tokyo
Nairobi Dar es Salaam Cape Town
Melbourne Auckland

and associated companies in
Beirut Berlin Ibadan Mexico City Nicosia

Oxford is a trade mark of Oxford University Press

Published in the United States
by Oxford University Press, New York

British Library Cataloguing in Publication Data
Haslam, Edwin
Metabolites and metabolism.
1. Metabolism, Secondary   2. Biosynthesis
3. Natural products
I. Title
574.19'29   QH521
ISBN 0-19-855377-3

Library of Congress Cataloguing in Publication Data
Haslam, Edwin.
Metabolites and metabolism.
Bibliography: p.
Includes index.
1. Metabolism, Secondary.   I. Title.
QH521.H37   1985   574.1'33   84-19040
ISBN 0-19-855377-3

Typeset by Joshua Associates, Oxford
Printed in Great Britain
at the University Press, Oxford
by David Stanford
Printer to the University

PREFACE

THE description 'natural product' is one readily recognized and comprehended by the organic chemist, for the roots of his science lie in the chemistry of 'natural products' and it evolved through the study of substances such as alkaloids, terpenes, and phenols isolated from plants and micro-organisms. In the early years of the twentieth century, theories began to be developed which aimed to suggest the probable origins of these 'natural products' from simple precursors. Their purpose was two-fold. Not only did they lay the foundations of biogenetic theory but they brought order and coherence to large groups of apparently unrelated 'natural products' by suggesting biochemical relationships. Biosynthetic experimentation over the past thirty years has sought to establish the validity of many of these biogenetic hypotheses. As the repertoire of methods has grown, then so has the subtlety and elegance of many of the investigations. Attention has shifted towards more intimate mechanistic details. Whilst such studies continue ('for that which often appears obvious, deserves and sometimes demands final proof') the pace of new discoveries in biosynthesis has slackened. Increasingly, investigators have begun to turn to the more biological problems which the presence of these 'natural products' or 'secondary metabolites' pose. As the distinguished natural products chemist T. A. Geissman predicted . . . 'the future . . . is to use the chemical information as the starting point for enquiry into questions that lie in the realms of biology'.

It is generally assumed that the metabolic capabilities of an organism must have been shaped by evolutionary processes, and as a consequence one of the most frequently-raised questions is that of the biological purpose or function of secondary metabolism and the selectionary advantage it has conferred. Before such questions can be properly approached, let alone answered, a great deal more requires to be learnt concerning the general biochemical matrix from which secondary metabolism derives, its enzymology, and the factors which operate to control and regulate secondary biosynthetic processes. Until such time, the debate concerning the possible role of secondary metabolism is likely to remain an inconclusive one.

Nevertheless, as a prelude to placing these metabolic events in a more precise biochemical context, the time is propitious to review our present knowledge of secondary metabolism. Whilst the text describes present views and ideas concerning four major groups of secondary metabolites—polyketides, alkaloids and amino-acid metabolites, plant phenols and terpenes, a detailed account of the biosynthesis of these 'natural products' has not been attempted. The text seeks rather to draw out some of the major themes of secondary metabolism, in a few instances some of its more subtle and intimate details, and finally its general biochemical characteristics as they have begun to emerge. Unsolved problems and those for the biologist to solve in the future are noted, and throughout the essential historical thread which links the unfolding story of 'natural product' biosynthesis from the eighteenth century to the present day is emphasized. As such, the text aims to attract both the chemist and the biologist by presenting a sufficiently detailed outline of both the framework of chemical ideas which surround the biosynthesis of 'natural products' and the numerous pertinent biological questions which surround the very presence of 'secondary metabolites' in plants and micro-organisms.

Sheffield   E. H.
March, 1984

For Rhodes and Hugh
Kelly

CONTENTS

1

INTRODUCTION

'We are like dwarfs on the shoulders of giants, so that we can see more than they . . . not by virtue of any sharpness of sight on our part, or any physical distinction, but because we are carried high and raised up by their giant size'.

Carl Wilhelm Scheele's scientific career was a brief one. His most important discovery, shared with Joseph Priestley, was undoubtedly that of the element oxygen, but this gifted Swedish chemist's other researches mark him, in a sense, as one of the founding fathers of Organic Chemistry. In the years 1769–85 he isolated, for the first time as crystalline substances, tartaric acid from grapes, citric acid [1.1] from lemons, malic acid [1.2] from apples, and gallic acid [1.3] from gall nuts.[1] Others were soon to add their own discoveries to those of Scheele such that Liebig's *Handbuch der Organische Chemie* of 1843 listed around 2000 substances derived from natural sources. The *raison d'être* for the development of organic chemistry as a scientific discipline can be traced to this point and to the desire of chemists to comprehend more fully these 'children of nature'. For over a century the elucidation of the chemistry of a natural product—its structure, chemical properties, and ultimately its synthesis—has been a dominant theme of organic chemistry. Today the emphasis has changed. These features of a natural product's chemistry which were once regarded as a sufficient end in themselves are now seen more as an indispensable prelude to a particular biological problem.

1.1. Secondary metabolism—definitions

With the flowering of the biochemistry in the twentieth century there came the realization that for many natural products (Fig. 1.1,*) a distinctive role in the life of organisms, whether they be microbes, plants, or mammals, could be assigned; fatty acids as components of lipid structures, α-amino-acids as building blocks of the ubiquitous proteins, and the heterocyclic purine and pyrimidine bases as units of nucleic acid structure which embody the genetic code.[2] Appropriately, two of Scheele's original discoveries—citric acid [1.1] and malic acid [1.2]—were themselves found to lie at the heart of carbohydrate metabolism as key intermediates of the Krebs, Citric Acid, or Tricarboxylic Acid Cycle. Natural products such as these occur in broadly similar patterns in most, if not all, organisms. The pathways by which they are synthesized are similar, if not identical in all organisms and these natural products are frequently referred to as

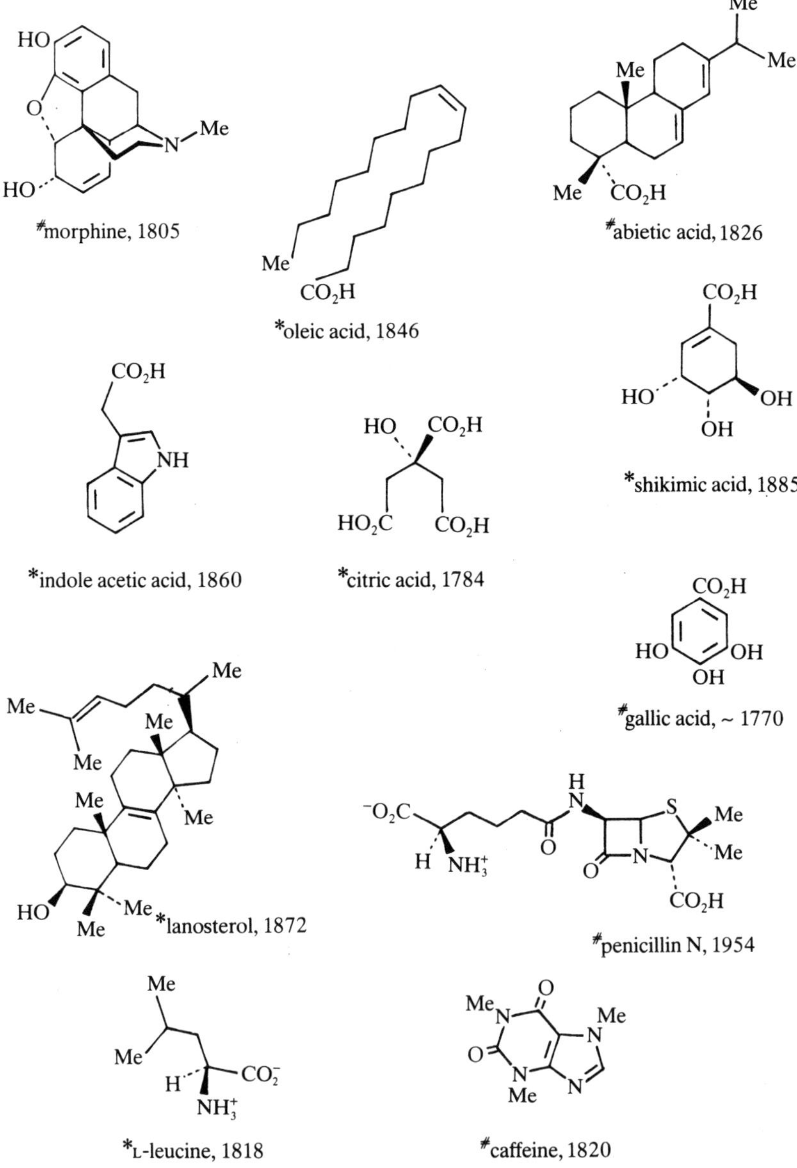

Fig. 1.1. Metabolites and metabolism.

primary metabolites. In contra-distinction, an infinitely greater body of natural substances—alkaloids, terpenes, polyenes, polyacetylenes, pigments, phenols, mycotoxins and so forth, occur sporadically throughout Nature and, moreover, they appear to have no explicit role in the welfare and economy of the producing organism (Fig. 1.1#).

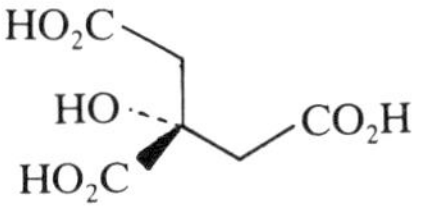

[1.1] 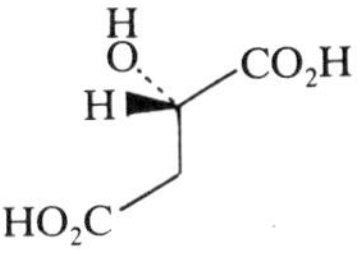   [1.2] 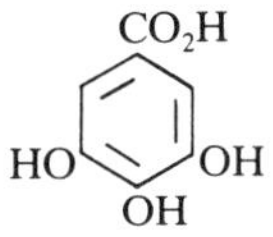   [1.3]

This distinction amongst natural products has long been recognized. Because of their apparently secondary role, the substances in this group are commonly referred to as secondary metabolites.[3] As Bu'Lock has remarked, they express the individuality of species in chemical terms. Whilst this discrimination between primary and secondary metabolism is useful in a didactic way, the boundary between the two areas of metabolism is nevertheless imprecise. Scientific opinions often differ as to the status of a particular metabolite, and as new discoveries are made then the boundary itself may change.

A few examples best illustrate the diffuse and ambiguous character of this division. Polyamines such as putrescine [1.4], spermine [1.5], and spermidine [1.6], and their biosynthetic enzymes, are ubiquitous in nature. They have a high affinity for DNA, stimulate protein synthesis, and microbial mutants exist in which there is a definite requirement of polyamines for growth. They have the aura of essential metabolites, and yet there is still no conclusive evidence to support any of their purported cellular functions. Similarly, scientific opinions may differ as to the status of a particular metabolite—especially those which are metabolically inert and have a restricted taxonomic distribution. Thus, the deposition of cellulose and the phenolic polymer lignin in plant cell walls is an essential phase in the development of the vascular character of plants. Both substances are metabolically inert, yet lignification is invariably referred to as a secondary process and lignin as a secondary metabolite.[3] Likewise carotenoids, because of their diversity of structural variation and distribution, have been referred to in the context of chemosystematics as secondary metabolites,[5] although many have clear, well-established functions in relation to photosynthesis and the survival of photosynthetic organisms. The differentiation in some cases

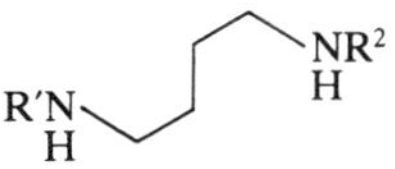

[1.4, R^1 = R^2 = H]
[1.5, R^1 = R^2 = (CH$_2$)$_3$NH$_2$]
[1.6, R^1 = H, R^2 = (CH$_2$)$_3$NH$_2$]

between primary and secondary metabolites may on occasion appear, if not illogical, then at least arbitrary. The reader should be aware of these uncertainties and that any particular classification may lack the imprimature of universal acceptance.

Bonner and Galston[3] recognized these difficulties which surround definitions based simply on the end-products of metabolic processes—the compound in isolation approach. Instead, they focused attention on the processes of metabolism and thereby distinguished 'the highways and byways' of metabolism. Those metabolic processes common to all forms of living matter, such as the synthesis and degradation of proteins, carbohydrates, and lipids are, by definition, the major highways. The byways are those processes by which chemical substances which are not apparently essential to the economy of the organism, are produced. There seems little doubt that, as Bonner and Galston implied, biochemical studies of secondary metabolism are ultimately best viewed in the context of the metabolic matrix in which they are enmeshed.

1.2　Biogenetic theories and biosynthetic pathways

Although it is only within the last thirty years, particularly with the advent of isotopic tracers and the techniques to monitor them, that progress has been made in the experimental study of the biosynthesis of natural products (secondary metabolites), the question of their origin in Nature has been one which has intrigued and preoccupied organic chemists for a great deal longer. Some, mistakenly perhaps, have described it as the last frontier of natural products chemistry. Whether one agrees with this description or not, the biosynthesis of natural products has provided a fertile field for both speculation and, later, experimentation. Eminent names—Robinson, Trier, Schöpf, Ruzicka, Barton, Collie, and Birch—were intimately associated with the initial formulation of hypothetical biogenetic pathways to natural products based upon *a priori* chemical reasoning. The exercise was both an intellectual challenge and a game. Those ideas which have stood the crucial test of time and which finally emerged from the pursuit of these inquiries form the body of *biogenetic theory*[3, 6].

The validity of many of these theories has been amply demonstrated. Not only have they formed the secure basis for the fruitful study of biosynthetic pathways *in vivo*, but they have been successfully employed as limiting factors in structure determination and, more recently, as aids to the design of laboratory syntheses of natural products—the so-called biomimetic synthesis, based on biogenetic analogy. Above all, they succinctly demonstrated how whole areas of natural product chemistry could be reduced from structural chaos to ordered array.[7]

Several strands of argument and reasoning contributed to the early development of biogenetic theories. First, there was the reasoning based on what has been aptly named 'comparative anatomy'. It was thus assumed that complex natural products are assembled from simpler molecules, which in turn are derived from common cellular metabolites. Recognition of these structural relationships provided the basis for much biogenetic speculation. The raw material for any biogenetic theory is a group of natural products through which runs some common and recognizable structural theme. Common structural features are then related to hypothetical biosynthetic precursors. The greater the number of structures that support the biogenetic concept the greater the confidence one may place in the idea. The isoprene rule and its derived biogenetic isoprene rule,[8] the acetate hypothesis[9] and comparative studies of alkaloid structures,[7] are outstanding examples of this approach to the study of biogenetic relationships amongst natural products. In addition, a major theme which underlines many of the more successful of these ideas was that Nature must work by laws recognizable to the chemist; the assertion that reactivities of the kind postulated in any biogenetic argument must be in accord with laboratory experience. As Robinson once remarked,[7] 'even enzymes are unlikely to disregard stereochemistry or the mode of electronic displacements in molecules'.

These theories provided the essential background for the experimental study of natural product biosynthesis. From this work there has emerged an elegant and eminently satisfying picture of the principal means whereby the main groups of natural products are synthesized *in vivo*. The biosynthesis of a great many natural products are now seen (Scheme 1.1) to proceed ultimately from just a few key intermediates of primary metabolism—phosphoenolpyruvate, pyruvate, acetyl coenzyme-A, 3-phosphoglycerate, oxaloacetate, and α-ketoglutarate, and principally (although not exclusively) α-amino acids synthesized directly from these intermediates (e.g. L-alanine) or by multi-step pathways from them (e.g. L-lysine and the aromatic amino-acids).

Nevertheless, despite these remarkable advances the picture of secondary metabolism is far from complete, for there is an inescapable logic behind the argument that to fully define metabolic pathways, study of the enzymes which catalyse each transformation is necessary. Probably because of the relative biochemical obscurity which secondary metabolites enjoy, and because of the technical difficulties involved, the enzymology of secondary metabolism is still in a fragmentary state. Until such time as this evidence becomes available, attempts, as suggested by Bonner and Galston, to place secondary metabolism in the context and framework of primary metabolism, are likely to be frustrated. Moreover, until these enzymological problems are clarified, it is clear that the insight provided by a shrewd chemical intuition will still continue to provide the most satisfactory rationale for the steps and sequences in many secondary pathways, and to shape the direction of future studies.

In this account of the principal routes of natural product biosynthesis, each area is developed from the point of view of the way in which the continual interplay of ideas and experiments has led to the present overall picture of the major events and pathways in secondary metabolism. Contributions from both

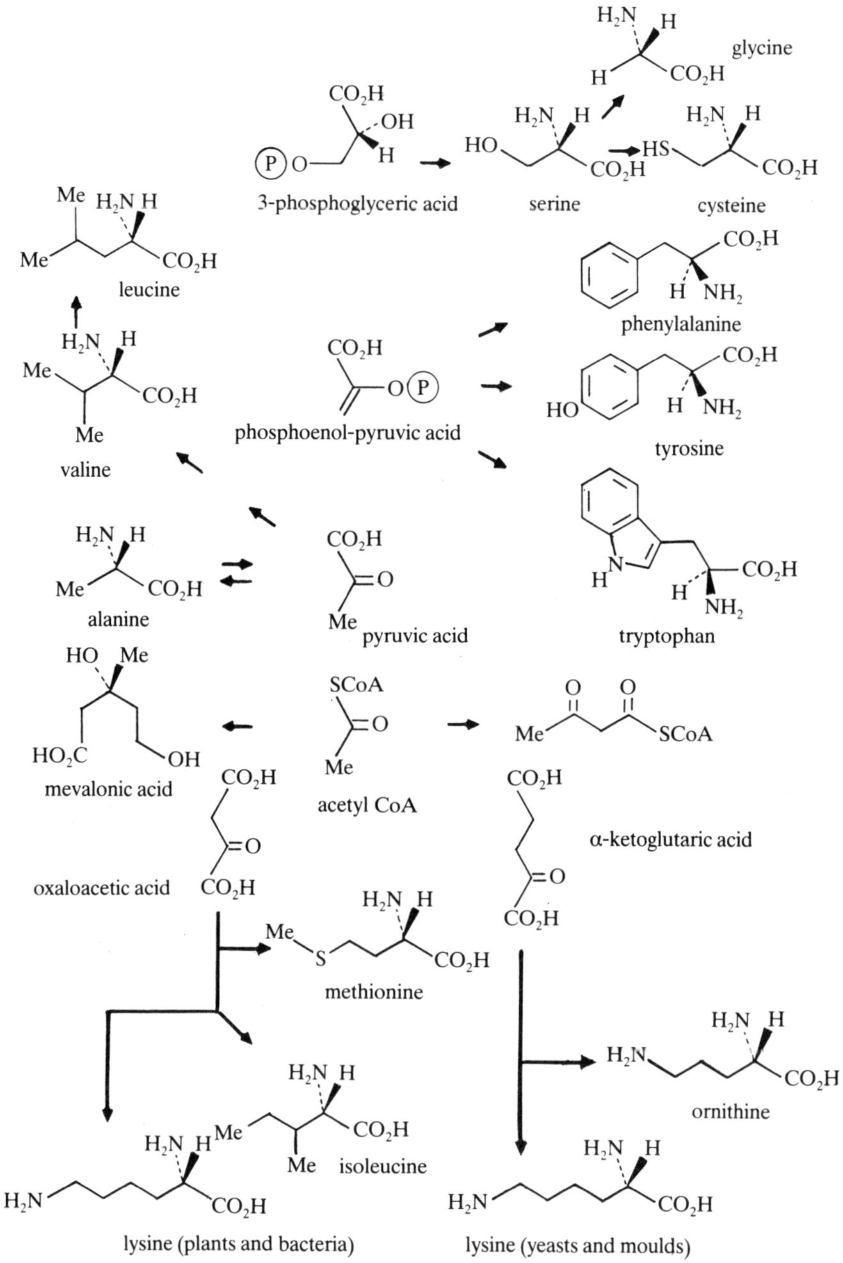

Scheme 1.1. Major intermediates in secondary metabolism.

theory and experiment are interwoven in the ensuing account. Some ideas have prevailed almost unchanged since their first introduction. Others have been modified, and some discarded, in order to account for particular experimental observations and increased general biochemical knowledge. Four broad fields are examined—polyketides, nitrogen-containing amino-acid derivatives, isoprenoids, and finally phenylpropanoid metabolites.

1.3 Methodology

Three general approaches have been used[10, 11] to study biosynthetic pathways and to obtain proof concerning biosynthetic intermediates:

   (i) the use of isotopically-labelled compounds as tracers;
   (ii) the use, *in vitro*, of extracted and purified enzyme systems; and
   (iii) the use, *in vivo*, of organisms with blocked biosynthetic pathways. The block may be endogenous and caused by a genetic mutation (e.g. auxotrophic microbial mutants) or it may be exogenous and induced by a chemical inhibitor.

While the evidence from each method, by itself, may be subject to diverse interpretations, the number of these can be considerably reduced by combining as many different approaches as possible. In practice, students of biosynthesis invariably rely on the single enzyme concept as the ultimate in positive evidence for particular steps and intermediates in a metabolic pathway. Thus, if a single enzyme can be shown to catalyse the conversion of A to B, and another single enzyme that of B to C, then compound B would satisfy the criterion of a true intermediate between A and C. The quality of the proof is limited solely by the reliability with which it is known that one is dealing with a 'single pure enzyme'. Difficulties in interpretation frequently involve metabolites, such as D in equilibrium with B. Here, steps A to D and D to C each require a mixture of two enzymes, and if homogeneity of the enzyme preparations cannot readily be established this may lead to erroneous conclusions.

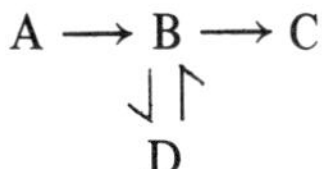

The study of the origins of secondary metabolites is one which falls broadly on the frontier between the province of the chemist and that of the biochemist. As such, it demands the knowledge and outlook of the biochemist, coupled with the chemist's intrinsic desire to rationalize the experimental observations within a satisfying and coherent chemical framework. Such hybrids are rare, and this has inevitably led to misunderstandings of the logical limitations of some of the methods employed. It is, for example, as Davis remarked in 1955, 'much easier to show that a compound can serve as a precursor of a cell constituent than to determine whether it is a normal, obligatory intermediate in the biosynthesis of that constituent'.

Until comparatively recently, much of the enzymatic machinery for secondary metabolites had proved remarkably inaccessible. Accordingly, the evidence for a great many of the pathways of secondary metabolism has relied heavily on the use of the isotopic tracer method [see (i) above]. Using this technique, bio-synthetic sequences are inferred after the administration of a putative inter-mediate or precursor, bearing one or more isotopic labels, to the intact organism or an enzyme preparation prepared therefrom. The end-product metabolite is then isolated and the position of the istopic label(s) determined. Incorporation of isotopically-labelled precursors may often be quite high in microbial experi-ments, whereas in higher plants, when often the whole plant has to be used, the yields are frequently rather modest. Indeed, as Cornforth has remarked,[12] 'It is surprising how many workers have tended to regard this appearance, in yields however miserable, as a sufficient demonstration'.

Isotopic tracer experiments in animals have often furnished critical proof that a particular substrate is an intermediate under physiological conditions, for it is possible to conduct such experiments without disturbing the substrate's con-centration in the body fluid. In plants and micro-organisms, by contrast, there is a greater burden of proof on the investigator to prove that under *normal* conditions of growth the cell actually utilizes the substrate in the prescribed manner.

Several variations of the straightforward tracer experiment may be executed. There is the technique of administering a labelled precursor and then examining the system to discover labelled substances other than the end-product that, from a chemical point of view, might be regarded as intermediates. Related thereto is the 'cold trap' experiment. Here, a suspected intermediate (unlabelled) is added to the system in which biosynthesis is in progress from an earlier (in the bio-synthetic pathway) labelled precursor. The suspected intermediate is re-isolated and analysed for isotopic label in the usual way. The concept was utilized, for example, by Bloch[14] to demonstrate that squalene [1.8] was an intermediate between acetate [1.7] and cholesterol (Scheme 1.2). He administered squalene to rats actively metabolizing 1-^{14}C-labelled acetate [1.7]. In this way he obtained specifically-labelled squalene [1.8] and then demonstrated that the radioactivity from this precursor was also incorporated into cholesterol [1.9].

Using the 'hot trap' experiment, a suspected intermediate labelled with one isotope is introduced into a system utilizing an earlier (biosynthetic) precursor with a different isotope. The incorporation of both isotopes into the end-product and of the precursor's isotope into the suspected intermediate, can be monitored in a single experiment. A typical example would be the addition of squalene labelled with tritium [^{3}H], [1.10], to a system metabolizing cholesterol from 1-^{14}C-acetate (Scheme 1.3). Doubly-labelled [^{14}C, ^{3}H] squalene and cholesterol [1.11] would then be isolated from the experiment.

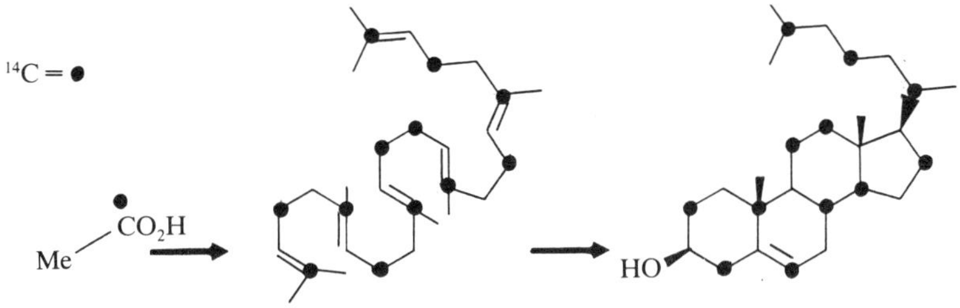

$^{14}C = \bullet$

$\underset{\text{Me}}{\overset{\bullet}{\diagup}}\!\!\text{CO}_2\text{H}$

[1.7]　　　　　[1.8, squalene]　　　　　[1.9, cholesterol]

Scheme 1.2. Biosynthesis of cholesterol: the 'cold trap'.

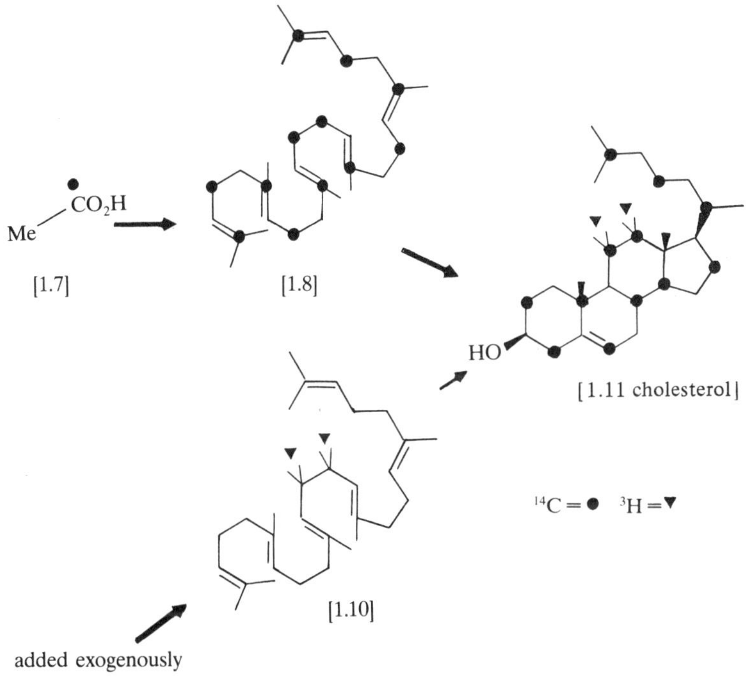

$\underset{\text{Me}}{\overset{\bullet}{\diagup}}\!\!\text{CO}_2\text{H}$

[1.7]　　　　　[1.8]

[1.11 cholesterol]

[1.10]

$^{14}C = \bullet \quad ^3H = \blacktriangledown$

added exogenously

Scheme 1.3. Biosynthesis of cholesterol: the 'hot trap'.

Successful application of the technique of sequential analysis depends upon a number of factors, not least the rate of enzymic synthesis of the sequence under investigation. The principle is succinctly illustrated by the method used to determine the direction of protein synthesis on the ribosome. Dintzis[15] employed a haemoglobin synthesizing extract, and analysed the soluble haemoglobin formed after pulse experiments with radioactively-labelled leucine. Peptides, derived by tryptic digestion of the protein, were analysed for radioactivity. After a short incubation, only peptides located near the carboxyl terminus contained radioactively-labelled leucine, but, as the incubation time increased, radioactivity was found progressively nearer to the amino terminus. Dintzis reasoned that protein molecules which contained labelled peptide fragments after short periods of incubation were those that had been nearly completed at the moment the isotopic tracer was added. To complete the synthesis of these protein molecules required the addition of just a few amino-acid residues (including leucine). Since, under these conditions, the radioactively-labelled fragments were found near the C-terminus it follows that this part of the polypeptide chain is synthesized last and grows linearly from the N-terminus.

When the technique is applied to the analysis of a biosynthetic sequence, a labelled precursor is added and the rate of appearance of the label into intermediates (W, Y, Z . . .) is analysed after different periods of metabolism (Scheme 1.4).

$$
\begin{array}{ll}
 & \overset{\bullet}{x} \\
 & \downarrow \\
t = o & x \longrightarrow w \longrightarrow y \longrightarrow z \\
t = a & \overset{\bullet}{x} \longrightarrow \overset{\bullet}{w} \longrightarrow y \longrightarrow z \\
t = b & \overset{\bullet}{x} \longrightarrow \overset{\bullet}{w} \longrightarrow \overset{\bullet}{y} \longrightarrow z \\
t = c & \overset{\bullet}{x} \longrightarrow \overset{\bullet}{w} \longrightarrow \overset{\bullet}{y} \longrightarrow \overset{\bullet}{z} \qquad \bullet\,\text{isotopic label}
\end{array}
$$

Scheme 1.4. Biosynthesis by sequential analysis.

A pertinent example of this approach in secondary metabolism is the work of Rapoport and his associates[16] on the opium alkaloids. After the administration of $^{14}CO_2$ as tracer, and a short period of metabolism, the ratio of specific activities of the alkaloids morphine [1.14] : codeine [1.13] : thebaine [1.12] was 5 : 77 : >300. After a prolonged period of metabolism (8 days) the ratio had changed to 463 : 346 : 200. The authors interpreted the results to show that biosynthetically thebaine [1.12] was first formed and then successively transformed by O-demethylation to codeine [1.13] and morphine [1.14]. Thus, if thebaine [1.12] was the earliest of the alkaloids to be synthesized, its specific activity would be the first to peak and the first to diminish.

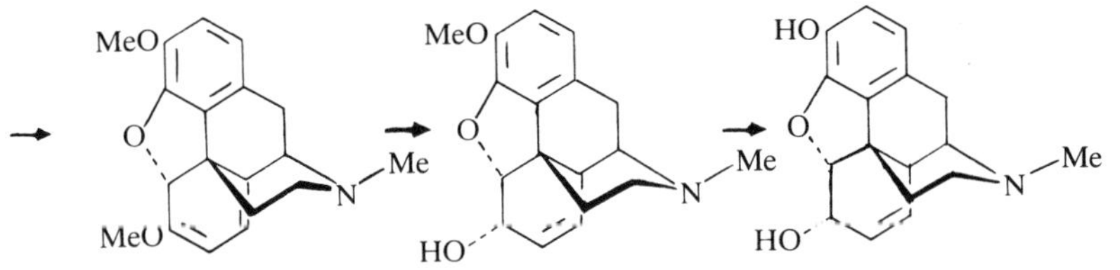

[1.12, thebaine]　　　　　[1.13, codeine]　　　　　[1.14, morphine]

Use of the isotopic tracer technique is nevertheless attended by several shortcomings and ambiguities in interpretation. Perhaps the two most serious of these are those of restrictive access, and aberrant synthesis (Scheme 1.5). In intact organisms, especially, the suspected biosynthetic intermediate may not penetrate to the site of synthesis due to permeability or transport problems (e.g. B, Scheme

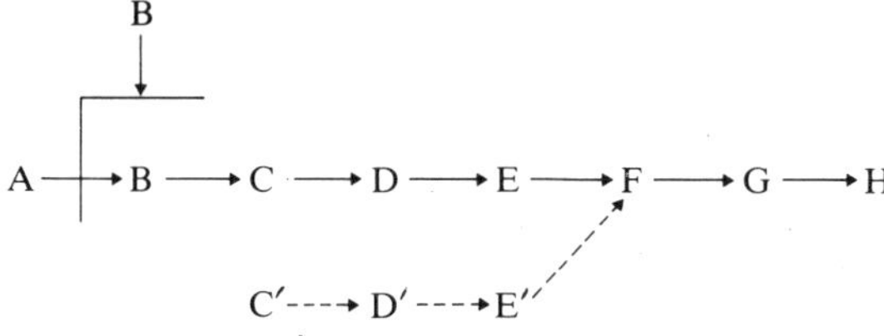

B — restricted acess
C′ — aberrant synthesis

Scheme 1.5. Restricted access, aberrant synthesis.

1.5), and a negative result in such circumstances may be entirely misleading. In other circumstances, a positive incorporation may again lead to quite erroneous conclusions. Thus, many enzymes of secondary metabolism as they have been characterized appear to have rather broad specificities, and in some cases substrates which resemble the biosynthetic intermediate may be metabolized by analogous pathways (e.g. C′, Scheme 1.5).

Whatever the perils of the isotopic tracer method, an essential feature of its use is the isolation and purification of the metabolite, and finally analysis to determine the position of the isotopic label(s).[13] The application of radioactive isotopes—particularly ^{14}C and ^3H—to label substrate molecules is now routine and it has enabled an imposing network of secondary metabolic pathways to be elaborated. The critical feature of the use of radioactive isotopes as tracers is the availability of unequivocal, high yield, chemical procedures to degrade the metabolite in order to isolate specific atoms in its structure. Often such degradations have to be carried through on a small scale and with low levels of radioactivity present.

Typical of the many biosynthetic investigations of this type is that carried out by Birch[17] and his colleagues with griseofulvin [1.15] an antibiotic metabolite of *Penicillium griseofulvum*. The molecule is a heptaketide and is derived by condensation of the biological equivalent of seven molecules of acetic acid.[9] With $1\text{-}^{14}C$ acetate [1.7] as precursor, griseofulvin [1.15] was isolated and degraded as shown in the annexed Scheme 1.6 to determine the positions of radioactively-labelled C-atoms—a remarkable and forbidding exercise!

Many biosynthetic reactions involve the addition of hydrogen to, or the removal of hydrogen from, a carbon atom, or the intramolecular transfer of hydrogen from one centre to another in a molecule. The intimate mechanistic detail of these processes are, in principle, susceptible to study with the two heavy isotopes of hydrogen—deuterium [^2H], whose presence or absence from a molecule may be determined by mass spectrometry or n.m.r., or the radioactive isotope tritium [^3H]. When used at virtually complete enrichment, deuterium is particularly well suited to the study of enzyme reactions *in vitro*. The attractions of deuterium diminish, however, when substantial dilution with unlabelled material occurs in the biochemical system under investigation (usually whole

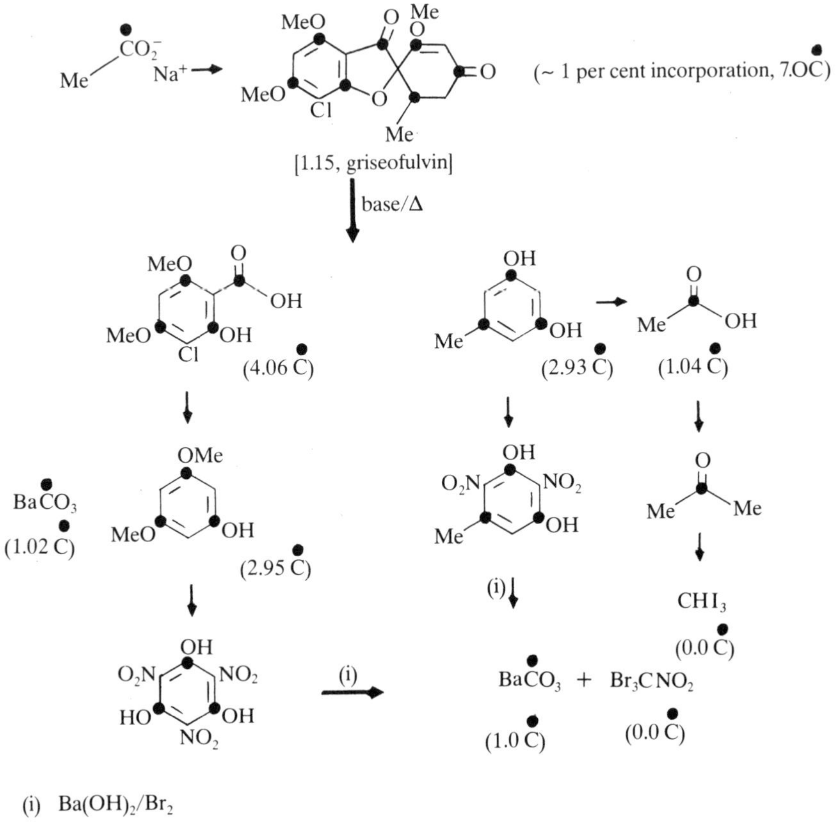

[1.15, griseofulvin]

(~ 1 per cent incorporation, 7.OC)

base/Δ

(4.06 C)

(2.93 C)   (1.04 C)

BaCO₃
(1.02 C)

(2.95 C)

(i)

CHI₃
(0.0 C)

BaCO₃ + Br₃CNO₂

(1.0 C)   (0.0 C)

(i) Ba(OH)₂/Br₂

Scheme 1.6. Biosynthesis of griseofulvin: degradation of the radioactive metabolite.

organisms). In these circumstances, tritium becomes the isotopic tracer of choice.

Some facets of their use as tracers may be seen in the study of the enzyme L-phenylalanine 4-hydroxylase[18] which catalyses the oxidative conversion of L-phenylalanine to L-tyrosine (Scheme 1.7). Using the 4-tritio substrate [1.16], a > 90 per cent retention of tritium was observed in the product [1.17] in the positions ortho to the introduced hydroxyl function—the so-called NIH shift. That this intramolecular transfer of hydrogen is subject to a kinetic isotope effect was neatly demonstrated, using the substrates [1.19] and [1.20], which showed a reduced tritium retention of just over 70 per cent, [1.18]. These observations led to the formulation of a mechanism for this reaction in which an oxepin intermediate [1.21] is formed, and in which the kinetic isotope effect is revealed in the final isomerization step (Scheme 1.7). Although this reaction was discovered and studied in relation to the metabolism of L-phenylalanine to the catechol amines in mammalian biochemistry, it is of fairly general occurrence and impor-

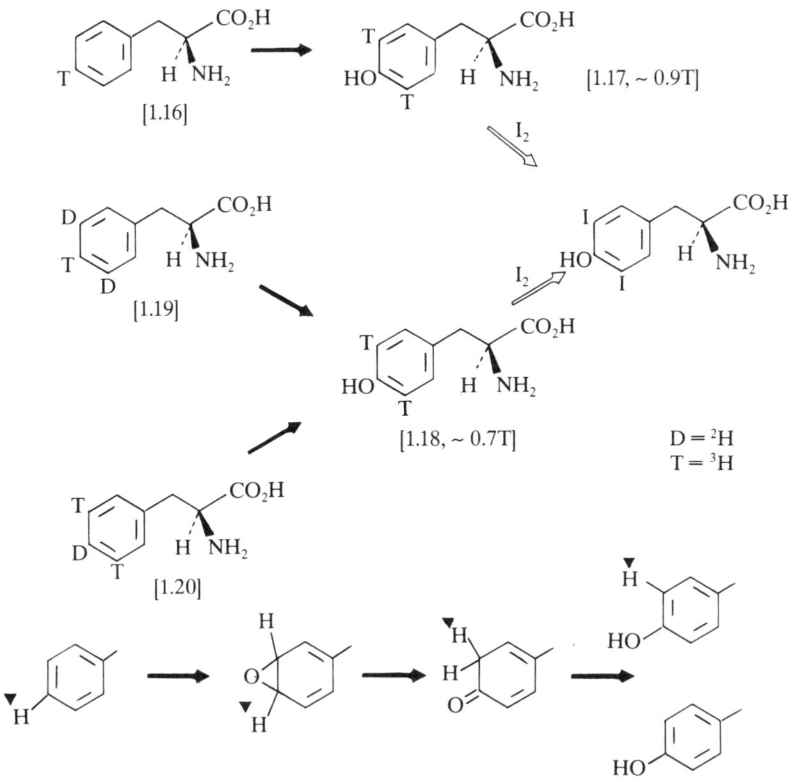

Scheme 1.7. L-Phenylalanine-4-hydroxylase: NIH shift.

tance in reactions which involve the hydroxylation of an aromatic ring. It is of apparently wide occurrence in aromatic secondary metabolism.

Advances in scientific knowledge frequently parallel advances in techniques and methodology consequent upon improved instrumentation. The use of ^{13}C n.m.r. in biosynthetic investigations is just such a case.[19] The major impetus to the introduction of this method was provided by the enhanced sensitivity which came with the development of pulse Fourier transform ^{13}C n.m.r. Isotopic tracer experiments using radioactively-labelled substrates usually require some chemical degradation procedure to determine finally the position(s) of the isotopic label. Such methods are time-consuming and frequently plagued with uncertainties.[13] Biosynthetic studies using ^{13}C n.m.r. to detect the ^{13}C isotope represents a genuine advance—particularly in microbial and *in vitro* enzyme studies—since the technique permits labelled atoms in a molecule to be located without degradation.

Successful application of the method generally requires:

(i) that the natural abundance ^{13}C n.m.r. spectrum of the metabolite can be unambiguously assigned;

(ii) that the incorporation of ^{13}C tracer is relatively good. Whilst very high incorporations can lead to problems of interpretation, to be detectable ^{13}C-enrichment should be at least 0.5–1.0 per cent above natural abundance (1.1 per cent); and

(iii) that dilution of the labelled precursor by a pool of unlabelled endogenous precursor is not such as to obscure the benefits of good incorporation.

The technique has found particular application in the study of the biosynthesis of microbial metabolites as for example polyketides—using 1-^{13}C, 2-^{13}C and 1, 2-^{13}C$_2$-acetate as precursors.[19] When doubly-labelled ^{13}CH$_3$.^{13}CO$_2$H [1.22] is used to label a microbial product of polyacetate origin, then the ^{13}C- ^{13}C couplings may be observed between the pairs of carbon atoms which are derived in the metabolite from the original C$_2$ acetate units. However, assuming incorporation is not too high, coupling should not be observed between adjacent C-atoms which are *not* derived from the same acetate unit, e.g. Scheme 1.8. Coupling constants are usually quite distinctive and diagnostic, and hence one can in this way delineate the position of intact acetate units in the natural product.

[1.22; 1,2-^{13}C$_2$-acetic acid]

6-methylsalicylic acid
^{13}C-^{13}C couplings
C-1 – CO$_2$H
C-2 – C-3
C-4 – C-5
C-6 – Me

Scheme 1.8. Biosynthesis of 6-methylsalicylic acid from, 1,2-^{13}C$_2$ acetic acid.

The simplicity and elegance of this method is amply illustrated by work on the mould metabolite griseofulvin [1.15] in *Penicillium urticae* (Scheme 1.9). Incorporation of 1-^{13}C acetate or 2-^{13}C acetate gave rise to a characteristic enhancement in the ^{13}C n.m.r. spectrum of griseofulvin of the signals from the appropriate carbon atoms (e.g. Scheme 1.6). When 1,2-^{13}C$_2$ acetate [1.22] was administered the ^{13}C n.m.r. spectrum of the derived metabolite showed ten pairs of coupled carbon atoms. Four pairs were readily discerned: C-1′ and C-3; C-2′ and C-3′; C-4′ and 5′ and C-6′ and C-Me. In the phloroglucinol ring A, however, six couplings were observed corresponding to all the possible combinations, e.g. C-3a and C-4 or C-3a and C-7a. To rationalize this observation it is assumed (Scheme 1.9) that the heptaketide cyclizes in stages, and that at an intermediate stage the benzophenone [1.23] is derived in a state which is not enzyme-bound. Free rotation around the aryl-carbonyl bond would then permit the metabolite derived from 1, 2-$^{13}C_2$ acetate to be composed of the two species [1.15*a*] and [1.15*b*]. This work contrasts neatly with the earlier methods of Birch, using ^{14}C as tracer (*vide supra*) and exemplifies once again the organic nature of science—the ability of later workers to build upon the observations of their predecessors.

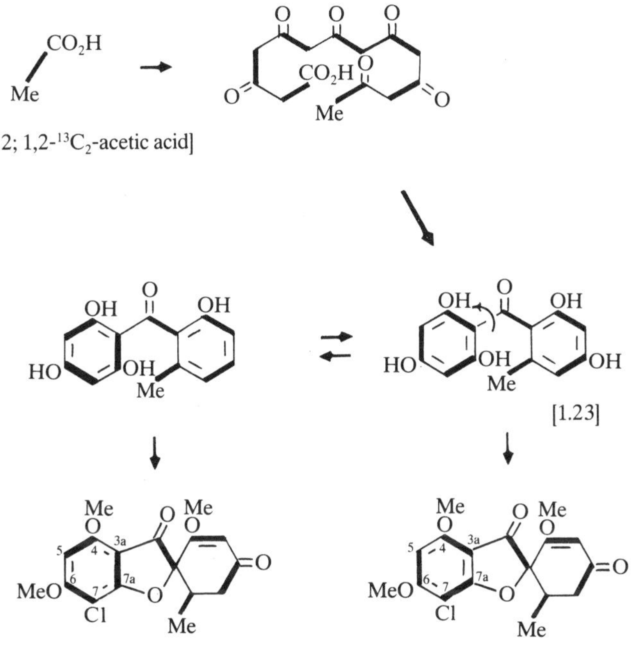

^{13}C-^{13}C couplings

[1.15*a*]	[1.15*b*]
C-3a – C-7a	C-7a – C-7
C-6 – C-7	C-5 – C-6
C-4 – C-5	C-3a – C-4

Scheme 1.9. Biosynthesis of griseofulvin [1.15] from 1,2-$^{13}C_2$ acetate.[20] (Two different couplings for each C-atom in phloroglucinol ring.)

References

1. PARTINGTON, J. R. *A history of chemistry*, vol. 3, pp. 205, 231. Macmillan, London (1962).
2. YUDKIN, M. and OFFORD, R. *Comprehensible biochemistry*. Longman, London (1973).

3. MANITTO, P. *Biosynthesis of natural products*, p. 9. Ellis Horwood, Chichester (1981).
   GEISSMAN, T. A. and CROUT, D. H. G. *Organic chemistry of secondary metabolism*. Freeman-Cooper, San Francisco (1969).
   BONNER, J. and GALSTON, A. W. *Principles of plant physiology*. Freeman-Cooper, San Francisco (1952).
4. BU'LOCK, J. D. in *Biosynthesis of mycotoxins* (ed. P. S. Steyn), p. 7. Academic Press, London and New York (1980).
5. LIAAEN-JENSEN, S. *J. pure & appl. Chem.* **51**, 661 (1979).
6. BU'LOCK, J. D. *The biosynthesis of natural products*. McGraw-Hill, London (1965).
7. ROBINSON, R. *The structural relationships of natural products*. Clarendon Press, Oxford (1955).
8. RUZICKA, L. *Proc. Chem. Soc.* 341 (1959).
9. BIRCH, A. J. *Proc. Chem. Soc.* 3 (1962).
10. ADELBURG, E. A. *Bact. Rev.* **17**, 253 (1953).
11. DAVIS, B. D. *Adv. Enzym.* **16**, 247 (1955).
12. CORNFORTH, J. W. *Chem. Soc. Rev.* **2**, 1 (1973).
13. BROWN, S. A. *Biosynthesis*, (ed. T. A. Geissman), Specialist Periodical Reports, Chemical Society, London, **1**, 000 (1972).
14. BLOCH, K. *Science* **150**, 19 (1965).
15. DINTZIS, H. M. *Proc. natn. Acad. Sci. U.S.A.* **47**, 247 (1961).
16. RAPOPORT, H., STERMITZ, F. R., and BAKER, D. R. *J. Am. Chem. Soc.* **82**, 2765 (1960).
17. BIRCH, A. J., MASSEY-WESTROP, R., RICKARDS, R. W., and SMITH, H. *J. Chem. Soc.* 800 (1958).
18. GOUROFF, G., DALY, J. W., JERINA, D. M., RENSON, J., WITKOP, B., and UDENFRIEND, S. *Science* **157**, 1524 (1967).
    KIRBY, G. W., BOWMAN, W. R. and GRETTON, W. R. *J. Chem. Soc. Perkin Transactions 1* 218 (1973).
19. MCINNES, G. A. and WRIGHT, J. L. C. *Acc. Chem. Res.* **8**, 313 (1975).
    SIMPSON, T. J. *Chem. Soc. Rev.* **4**, 497 (1975).
    SCOTT, A. I. *Science* **186**, 101 (1974).
20. SATO, Y. and ODA, T. *Tetrahedron Lett.* 3971 (1976).

2

POLYKETIDES AND THE ACETATE HYPOTHESIS

2.1 Introduction

The polyketides are a group of natural products which were first defined as a result of comparative structural analysis and correlation.[1] They are of importance in both plants and micro-organisms, and encompass a wide range of substances such as phenols, quinones, xanthones, flavonoids, and numerous mycotoxins. Their structures perfectly illustrate one of the outstanding general features of secondary metabolism, namely the apparent biosynthetic prodigality of organisms; endless variations appear to be elaborated on one major chemical theme. Variety is engendered within a single structural grouping by the multiple branching of synthetic pathways which are frequently oxidative in character. A plausible explanation of this general characteristic is that an accumulation of intermediates is built up in some primary pathway, and that enzymes are then activated or induced for the synthesis of secondary metabolites from one or more of these primary products. Frequently, one key secondary metabolite is envisaged as being formed, and this then undergoes a wide range of chemical changes leading to a spectrum of secondary products, each one only slightly different from the rest. Such schemes and patterns may embrace a multiplicity of pathways, although only one of these may well be expressed in a particular plant or micro-organism.

2.2 The acetate hypothesis

The impetus for the acetate hypothesis, which embraces the biosynthesis of polyketides, derived largely from attempts to extrapolate the known biochemical significance of acetic acid, as a building unit in fatty acids and steroids, to phenolic and enolic systems. In particular, it was postulated that the oxygen atoms retained in the metabolite might reflect its origin from acetic acid, and, moreover, they might be used as markers to identify the position of carboxyl carbon atoms of acetic acid units in the structure of a secondary metabolite. When Birch initiated his work, it was known that fatty acids were formed by the head-to-tail linkage of acetic acid units. At each condensation step the carbonyl group is reduced and the oxygen atom eliminated by dehydration. Reduction finally converts the original carbonyl group to methylene (Fig. 2.1). The acetate hypothesis was based primarily on a consideration of what might happen if the β-oxygen atoms were not serially reduced out, and instead a β-polyketomethylene system was formed as its terminal coenzyme A ester [2.1]. Some time after the announcement by Birch of the acetate hypothesis, it became clear that although acetyl coenzyme A is the 'starter' unit in fatty acid biosynthesis the 'chain extension' unit is malonyl coenzyme A, formed by carboxylation of acetyl coenzyme A (Scheme 2.1).

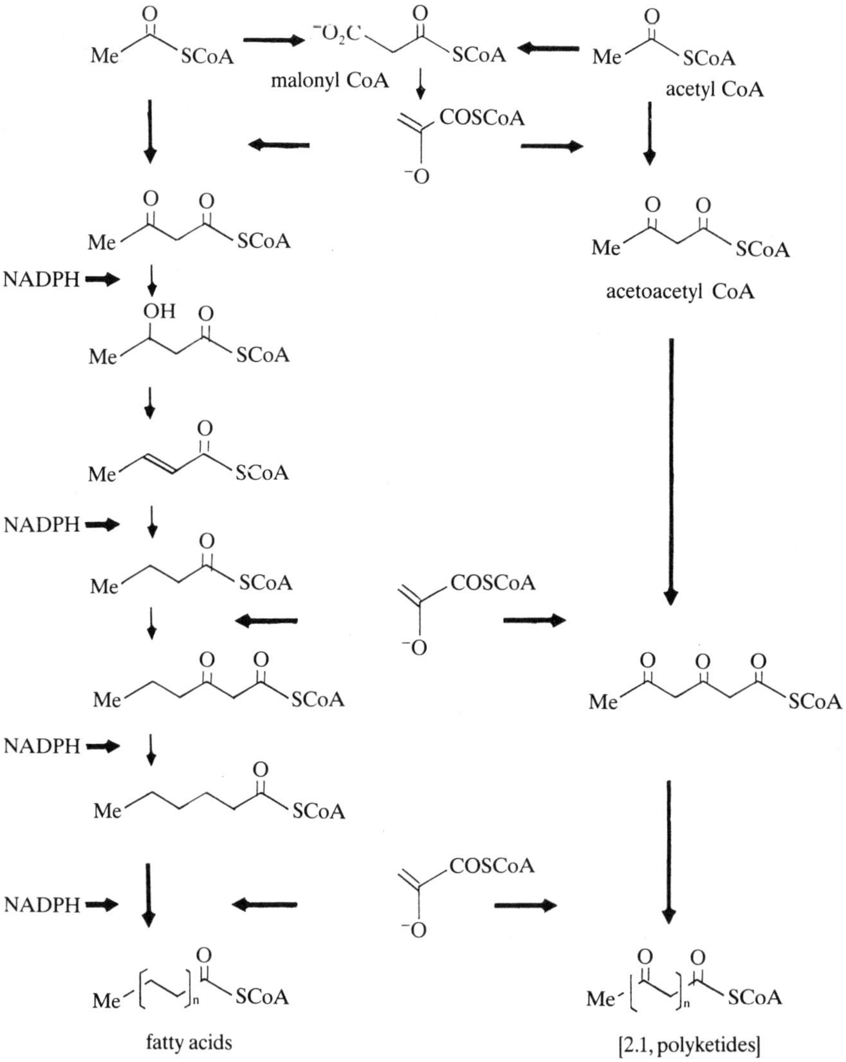

Scheme 2.1. Fatty acid and polyketide metabolism.

One of the most compact groups of natural products which had been shown to be ultimately derived from acetic acid, and consideration of which originally laid the foundations for the acetate hypothesis, are the depsides and depsidones derived from orsellinic acid [2.2][1] The depsides (e.g. evernic acid, [2.3]) are simply esters of two or more orsellinic acid-type units. In an examination of

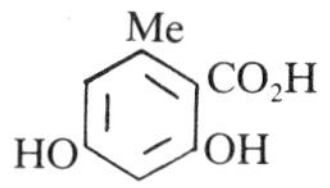

[2.2; orsellinic acid] 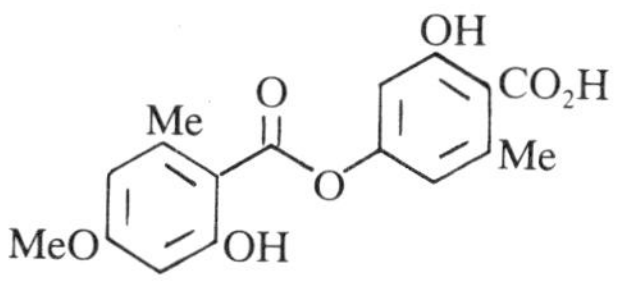   [2.3; evernic acid]

the units obtained by the hydrolysis of the depside ester bond of a group (thirty) of lichen didepsides and tridepsides, they were all shown to have the form depicted in formula [2.4], in which $n = 1, 3, 5,$ or 7. The side chain (C_n) at position 6 always has an odd number of carbon atoms. Substituents at the 3 and 5 positions are less numerous and, unlike those at the 1, 2, 4, and 6 positions, can be either one carbon, or oxygen, and occasionally halogen substituents.

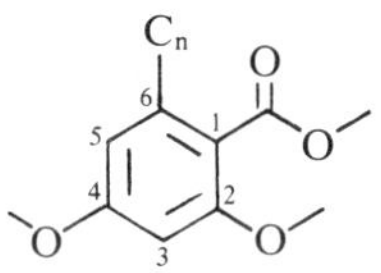

[2.4]

Statistical analysis of structures, structural comparisons, and correlations of this type amongst a whole range of natural products besides depsides, such as xanthones, acetophenones and phloroglucinol derivatives, flavonoids, naphthoquinones, and anthraquinones, led Birch to suggest that these secondary metabolites were formed wholly, or in part, from β-polyketomethylene chains which were in turn assembled by head-to-tail linkage of acetic acid units. Orsellinic acid (Scheme 2.2) [2.2], it was thus proposed, was derived in the manner shown by cyclization of a β-tetraketide chain.

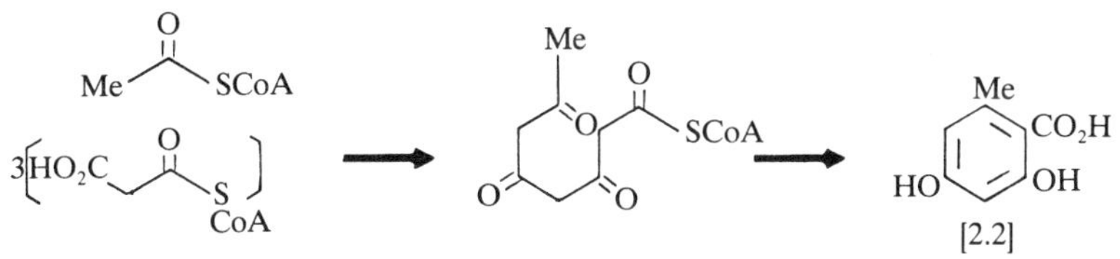

[2.2]

Scheme 2.2. Biosynthesis of orsellinic acid.

Fig. 2.1. Some polyketide metabolites.

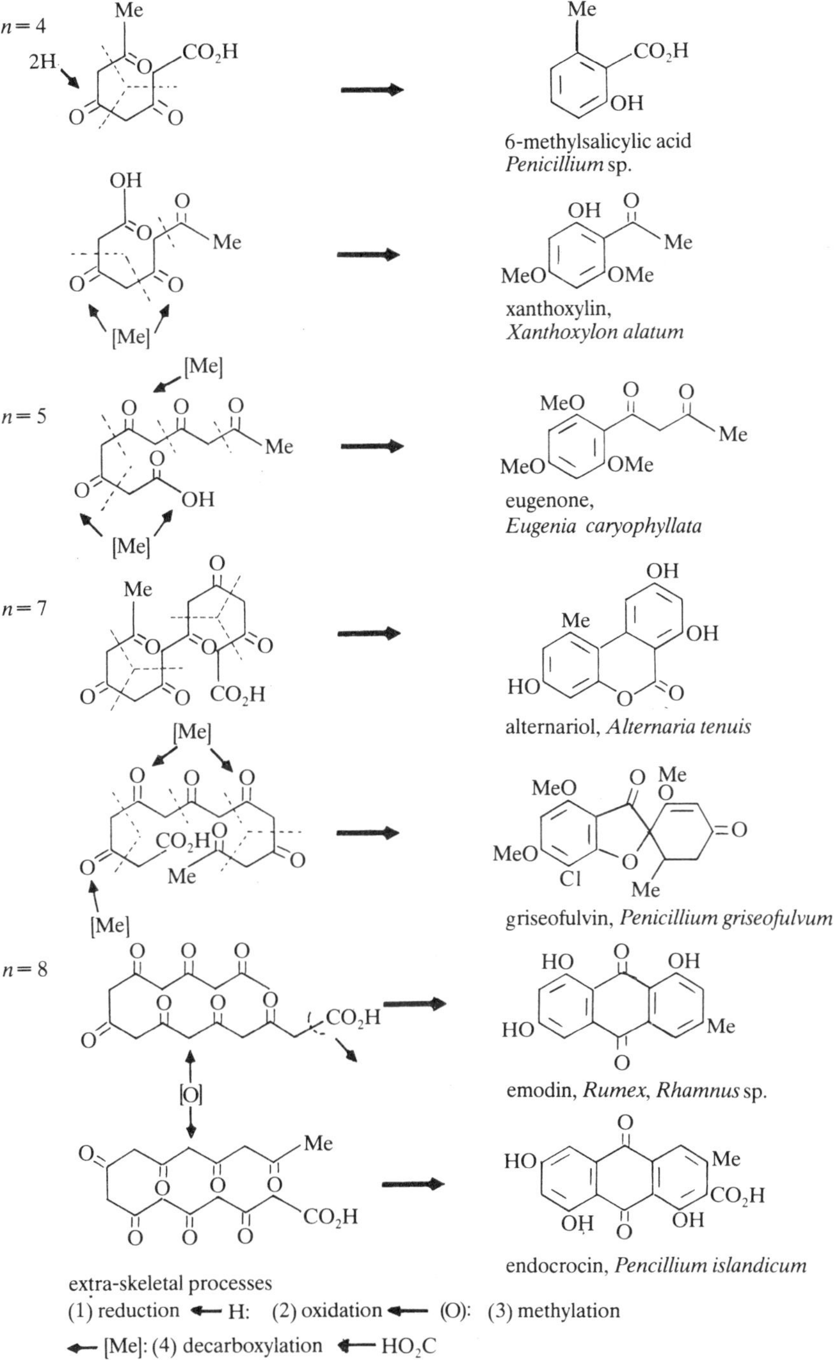

Fig. 2.1. Continued.

The timing of Birch's exposition of the acetate hypothesis was propitious, since the isotopic tracer techniques appropriate for the experimental testing of these ideas were just beginning to be employed. It is, however, worth recording that Collie had put forward the bones of a similar hypothesis in 1907 based on the condensation and cyclization of synthetic β-polyketones.[2] Unfortunately, it was neglected, and exercised little influence on thinking in these areas in the intervening period of nearly fifty years.

The basic concepts underlying the acetate hypothesis are very few and of 'an engaging simplicity'. The theory requires the following assumptions:

(a) Acetic acid units are joined by the formal elimination of water in head-to-tail linkage with each other or with other naturally-occurring carboxylic acids to form β-polyketomethylene chains.

(b) These β-ketomethylene chains may undergo secondary changes: notably they may cyclize by reactions of the Claisen or Aldol type to form aromatic rings.

(c) The carbon skeleton so formed may be modified by the introduction of alkyl groups (e.g. methyl, isopentenyl).

(d) Secondary processes of reduction (sometimes accompanied by dehydration) and of oxidation may occur either before or after cyclization.

Once the rules have been correctly assimilated they are, with a little imagination, easy to apply as an exercise in 'paper chemistry'.

The nature of the final products depends on the carboxylic acid which initiates the synthesis, the number of acetic acid units involved (the size of the polyketide), the mode of ring closure, and the nature and number of modifying substituents and reactions which seem to embroider, in a chemical sense, the final structure. Figure 2.1 shows selected examples of natural products of plant and microbial origin which conform wholly, or in part, to the fundamental tenets of the acetate hypothesis.

Many natural substances are, for example, directly derived, without further modification, by simple cyclization of a poly-β-ketomethylene chain (e.g. Figure 2.1, pinocembrin, orsellinic acid, alternariol). Others are very closely related to those lying within the direct scope of the theory, but they may lack expected carboxyl groups (e.g. Fig. 2.1, pinosylvin, emodin), or oxygen atoms (e.g. Fig. 2.1, piperine, kawain, hydrangeol, 6-methyl-salicylic acid). Others contain additional oxygen atoms—usually as phenolic hydroxyl or quinonoid oxygen —(e.g. Fig. 2.1, emodin, endocrocin), or additional alkyl groups such as methyl, isopentenyl, dimethylallyl (e.g. Fig. 2.1, kawain, anibine, xanthoxylin, eugenone, griseofulvin). The removal of oxygen is believed to involve reduction of a carbonyl group in a non-aromatic precursor followed by dehydration. Similarly, the addition of oxygen *ortho* or *para* to an existing hydroxyl function in an aromatic ring is chemically feasible and has good chemical analogies. Alkylation is again chemically acceptable *ortho* or *para* to a phenolic group if the alkylating agent is electrophilic in character. Later biochemical work has shown methylation frequently to occur *via* the agency of S-adenosyl methionine ([2.5] SAM) and the C_5 terpenoid groups are most probably introduced via dimethylallyl pyrophosphate [2.6].

[2.5; S-adenosyl methionine]

[2.6, DMAPP]

2.3 Sequences and the timing of steps

Robinson in his theories of alkaloid biogensis described these subsidiary processes, such as methylation, oxidation, and decarboxylation, as *extra-skeletal*, and he suggested that they might be considered to occur at any convenient stage of an assumed biosynthetic pathway. As techniques to study secondary biosynthesis have advanced, then so the question of the timing of these extra skeletal processes has assumed a greater importance. Some, for example O-methylation in phenolic systems, are clearly critical in determining subsequent stages of the pathways of metabolism. Some of these subtleties are revealed by work with griseofulvin, a mould metabolite.[4] Griseofulvin [2.7] is a chlorine-containing antibiotic elaborated by *Penicillium griseofulvum* and other *Penicillia sp.* As it is presently understood, the biosynthesis of griseofulvin involves the cyclization of a poly-β-ketomethylene chain intermediate of seven acetic acid units to a benzophenone, followed by intramolecular oxidative coupling to give the grisan structure. Co-metabolites of griseofulvin include the benzophenone derivaties ([2.8] [2.9] [2.10]; griseophenones, A, B, and C) and dehydrogriseofulvin [2.11]. The timing of the methylation and chlorination steps have been studied by the classical tracer techniques (see Chapter 1), whereby putative intermediates are labelled with one or more isotopes and administered to the organism. If the substrate is a precursor, then the content and position of isotopic species in the metabolite should be directly related to those of the substrate.

Dehydrogriseofulvin [2.11] is thus efficiently transformed into griseofulvin [2.7], and griseophonones C [2.10] and B [2.9] can similarly be demonstrated as sequential intermediates on the biosynthetic pathway. Griseophenone A [2.8] does *not* act as a precursor of griseofulvin. More recent studies have similarly shown the grisan [2.12] to be a precursor of griseofulvin and [2.13] to be the first O-methylated benzophenone on the pathway. For these studies, the grisan [2.12] was prepared labelled with ^{14}C by chemical transformation of griseofulvin biosynthesized from 1-^{14}C-sodium acetate (Fig. 2.2). The benzophenone [2.13] was prepared by direct chemical synthesis bearing the O-methyl group labelled with tritium (^{3}H) (Fig. 2.3).

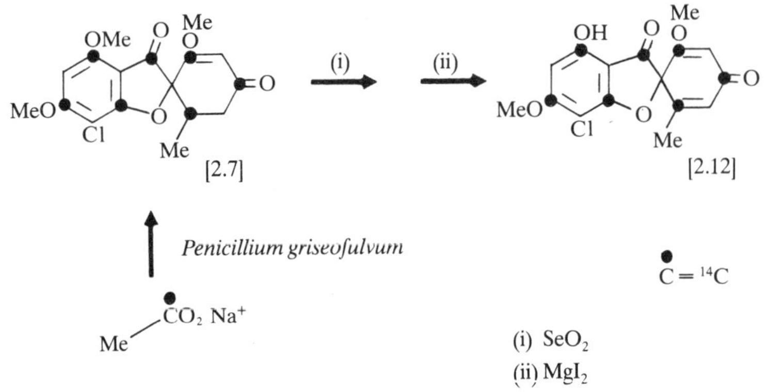

Fig. 2.2.

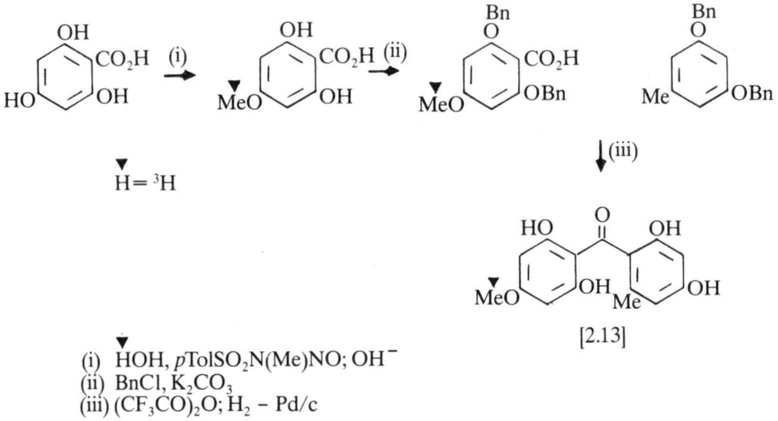

Fig. 2.3.

In a similar vein, mycophenolic acid [2.14] is a metabolite of *Penicillium brevicompactum*.[5] The phthalide nucleus is acetate-derived and the attached carbon chain is isoprenoid in origin. Tracer experiments with ^{14}C-methionine [2.15] provided the first experimental proof of biological C-methylation in the synthesis of a secondary metabolite. Orsellinic acid [2.2] is *not* an intermediate and the C-methylation process has been postulated to occur at the stage of the poly-β-ketomethylene precursor, presumably via an enol form (Scheme 2.4).

2.4 Oxidative transformation of polyketides

Griseofulvin [2.7] and mycophenolic acid [2.14] exemplify the fact that in some organisms the range of metabolites obtained via the cyclization of poly-β-ketomethylene precursors is considerably enhanced and diversified by further transformations—frequently oxidative in character—which may occur. In *Penicillium cyclopium*, for example, a series of anthraquinone derivatives based on emodin are found. These differ [2.16, *a, b, c, d*] only in the state of oxidation of a one-carbon substituent, and suggest that the pathway Me→CH$_2$OH→CHO→CO$_2$H is a common biosynthetic sequence.

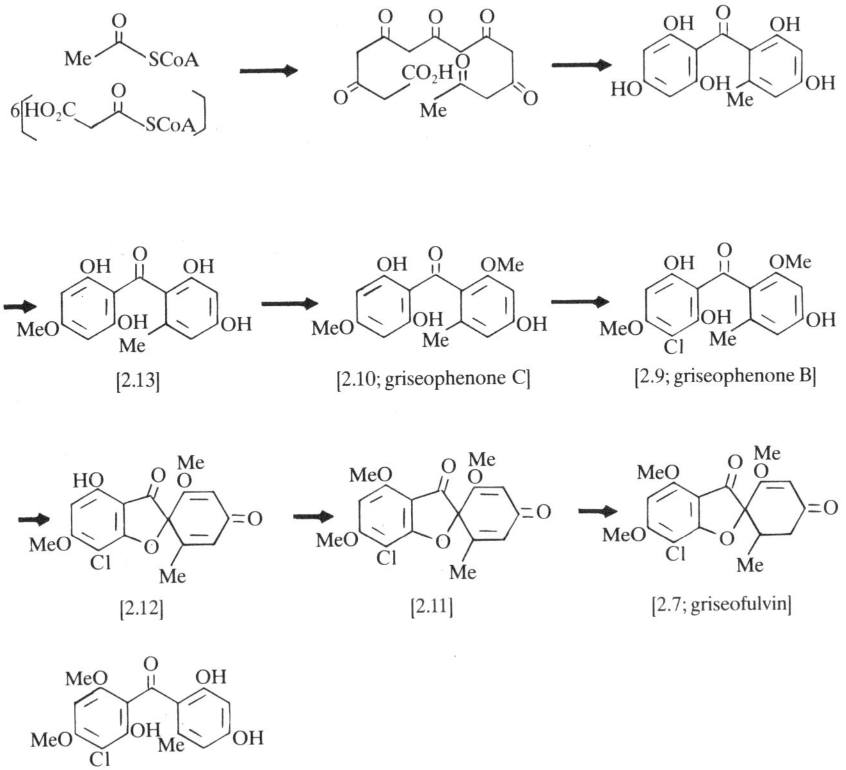

[2.13]   [2.10; griseophenone C]   [2.9; griseophenone B]

[2.12]   [2.11]   [2.7; griseofulvin]

[2.8; griseophenone A]

Scheme 2.3. Biosynthesis of griseofulvin.[4]

The oxidative coupling of phenolic nuclei is another important biosynthetic process encountered in polyketide and other areas of metabolism.[6] Several enzyme systems are known which will bring about the oxidation of phenols, and good laboratory analogies are provided by a range of inorganic oxidants such as ferric chloride and potassium ferricyanide. It is customary (although not obligatory) to formulate such reactions as one-electron oxidations of the phenolate anion. Formation of the grisan structure in griseofulvin biosynthesis is typical of these phenolic coupling reactions (Scheme 2.5).

Historically, the most eloquent demonstrations of the importance of phenolic coupling in the development of biogenetic theory were Robinson's proposals[3]

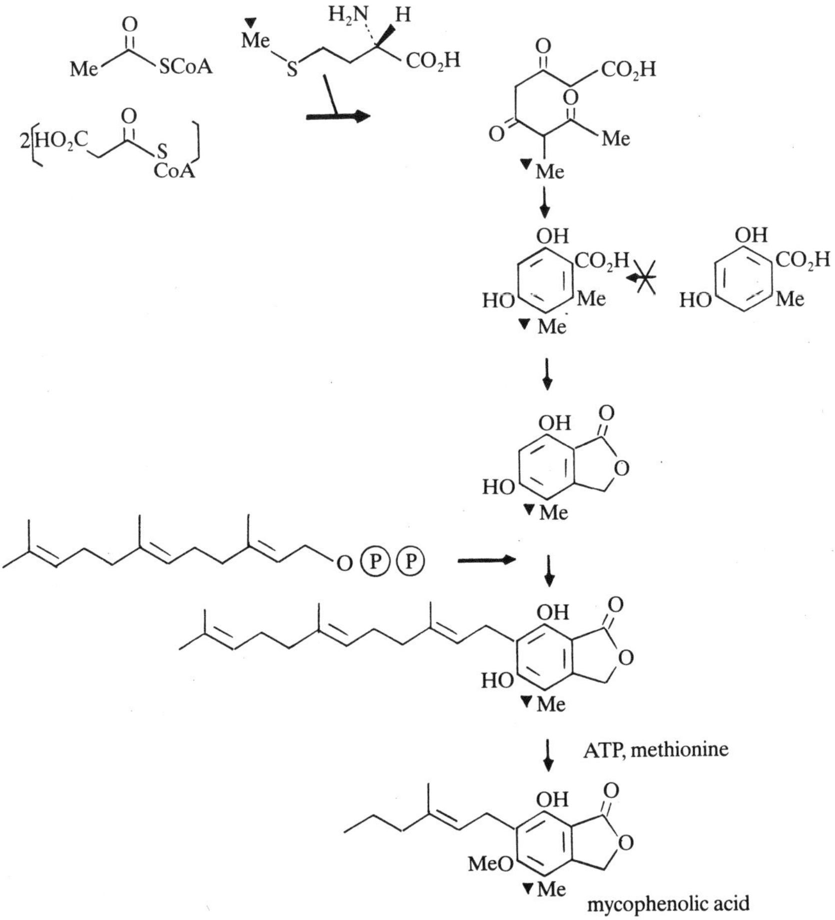

Scheme 2.4. Biosynthesis of mycophenolic acid.[5]

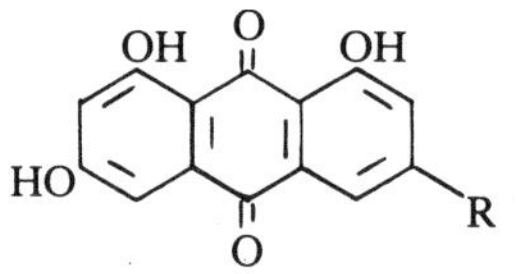

[2.16*a*, R = Me: emodin]
[2.16*b*, R = CH$_2$OH]
[2.16*c*, R = CHO]
[2.16*d*, R = CO$_2$H]

to relate the structures of the morphine–thebaine group of alkaloids to those of the other opium bases, and Barton's suggestions concerning the biogenetic origin of the phenol usnic acid [2.17] in the lichen *Usnea diffracta*.[6] The key step in the biosynthesis of usnic acid, Barton recognized as the oxidative coupling of two molecules of methylphloracetophenone [2.18] (Scheme 2.6). An elegant biomimetic synthesis of usnic acid was modelled on this hypothesis using potassium ferricyanide as the *in vitro* oxidant.

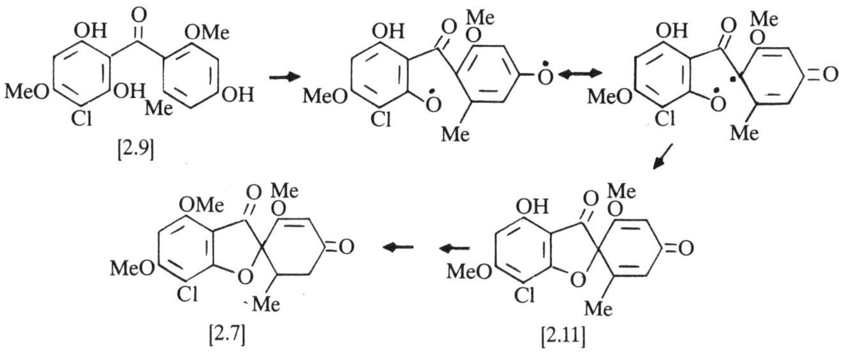

[2.9]

[2.7] [2.11]

Scheme 2.5. Phenolic coupling in griseofulvin biosynthesis.

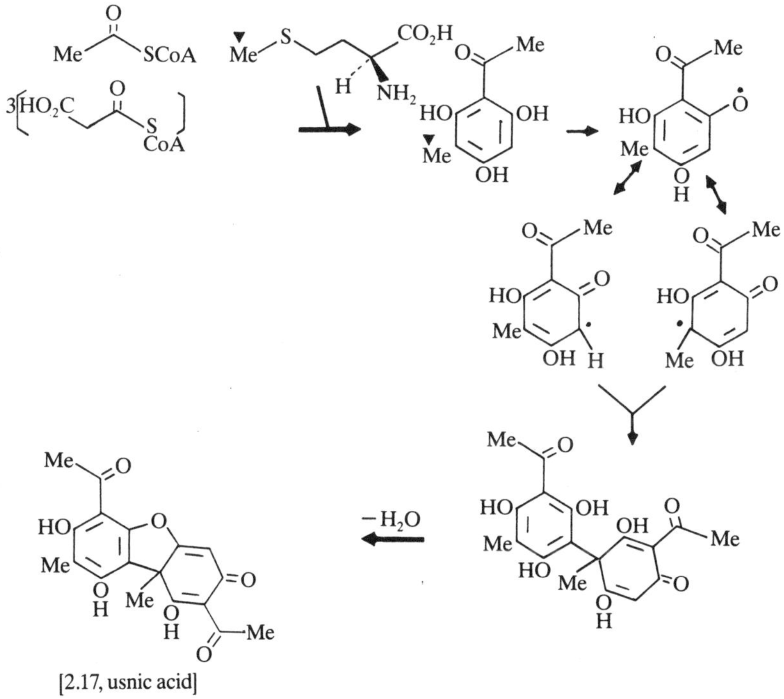

[2.17, usnic acid]

Scheme 2.6. Biosynthesis of usnic acid.[6]

In the examples of polyketide metabolites discussed up to this point, the origins of the secondary product from acetate is generally discernable, either wholly, or in part, from an inspection of the structure. However, for several secondary metabolites the original polyketide undergoes more deep-seated structural reorganization, usually as a result of oxidative transformations such that the final structure no longer resembles that of a polyketide. Typical examples are: the formation of penicillic acid [2.19] from orsellinic acid [2.2] in *Penicillium cyclopium*, patulin [2.20] from 6-methyl salicylic acid [2.21] in *Penicillium patulum*, and stipitatonic acid [2.22] from 3-methylorsellinic acid [2.23] in *Penicillium stipitatum*. In each case the structural change is believed to follow oxidative aromatic ring fission.[7] A possible pathway is suggested for the formation of penicillic acid (Scheme 2.7).

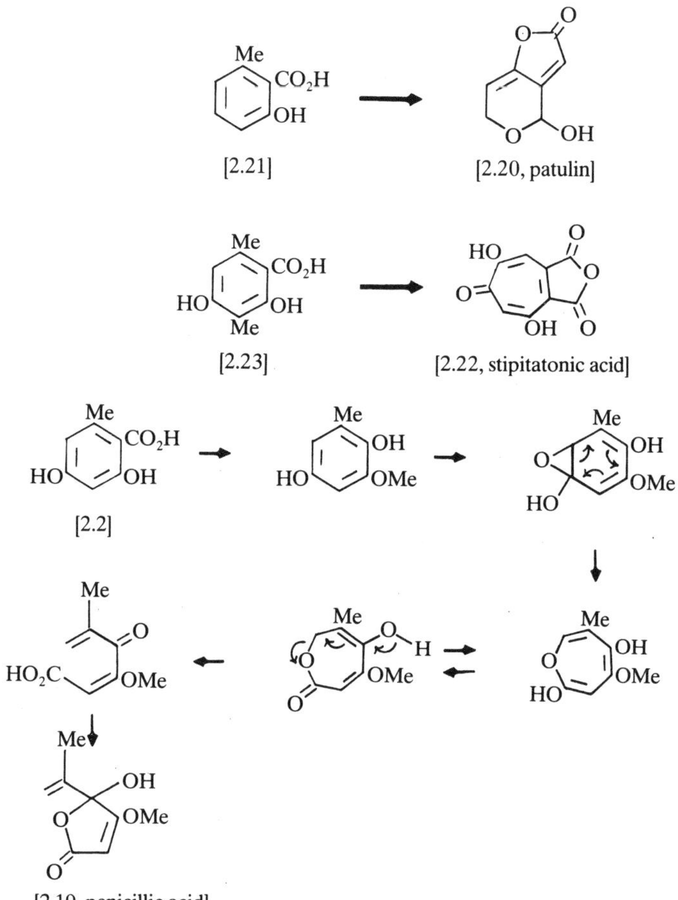

Scheme 2.7. Ring fission in polyketide biosynthesis.[7]

The apotheosis of this type of structural reorganization consequent on the formation of the first aromatic metabolite is probably represented[8] by the biosynthetic pathway to aflatoxin B-1 [2.24]—a potent mycotoxin of *Aspergillus flavus* (Scheme 2.8).

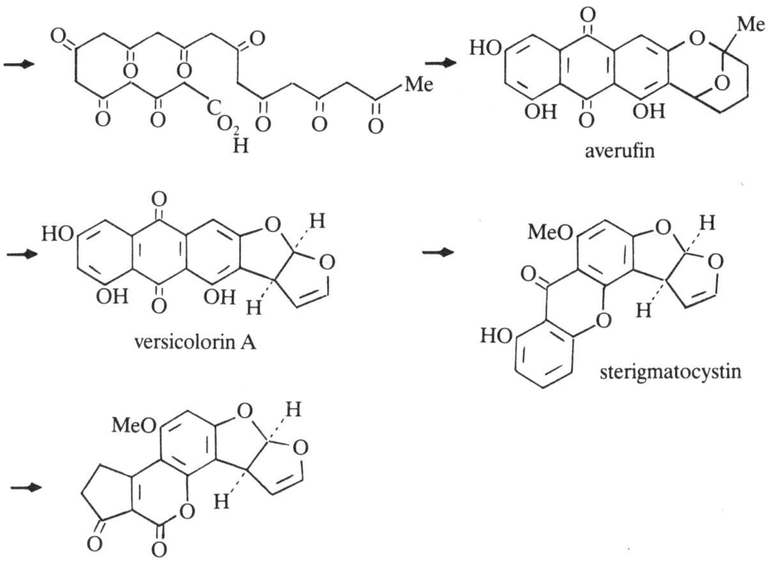

averufin

versicolorin A

sterigmatocystin

[2.24, aflatoxin B-1]

Scheme 2.8. Proposed biosynthetic pathway to aflatoxin B-1.[8]

2.5 Polyketides derived from other acids

Although the acetate hypothesis was originally devised to rationalize the biogenetic origins of a wide range of natural products from the C_2 acetate unit,
subsequent work has shown that several fungal metabolites are derived by the
assembly, wholly or in part, of C_3 and C_4 carboxylate units. Important groups
of substances which fall into this category are the ansamycin[9] and the macrolide
antobiotics.[10] Natural macrocyclic lactones (macrolides) are divisible into several
classes according to their biogenetic origins:

    (i) those derived entirely from propionate, C_3;
   (ii) those derived from acetate (C_2) and propionate (C_3); and
  (iii) those derived from acetate (C_2), propionate (C_3), and butyrate (C_4),
       or its biological equivalent.

The erythromycins are a classic example of the first group. Tracer and mutant
studies have shown that the macrocyclic ring is synthesized from seven propionate units (a starter unit of propionyl CoA and six methylmalonyl CoA
extension units). A typical example is erythromycin A [2.25] (Scheme 2.9).
In contrast, the ansa-bridge of rifamycin B [2.26] is derived from both acetate
and propionate units (Scheme 2.9).

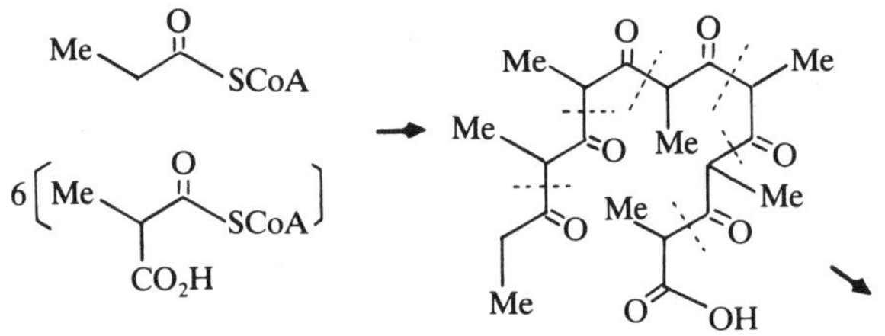

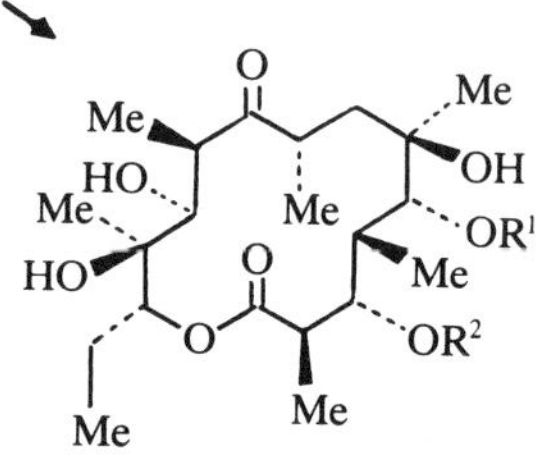

[2.25], R^1 = desosamine
R^2 = cladinose
erythromycin A,
(*Streptomyces erythreus*)

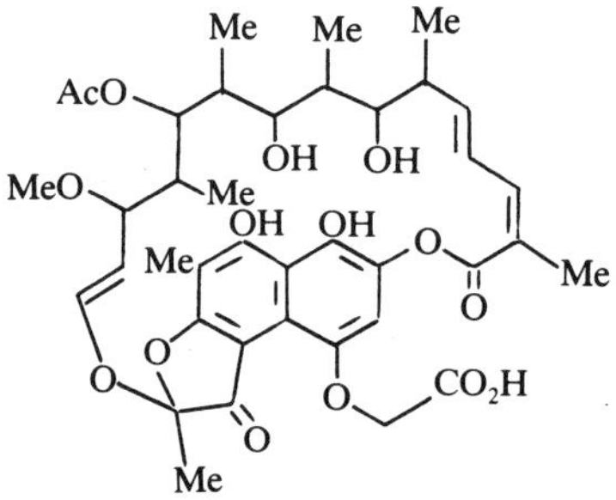

[2.26, rifamycin B]

Scheme 2.9. Mixed polyketides.[9, 10]

2.6 Unresolved questions

Two points of continued uncertainty in polyketide biosynthesis and to which clear answers are not yet possible are:

(i) to what extent are the processes of chain assembly and cyclization distinguishable?

(ii) what are the factors which determine the overall mode of cyclization of the β-ketomethylene chain?

The multi-enzyme complex—6-methylsalicylic acid synthetase—which catalyses the conversion of acetyl coenzyme A and malonyl coenzyme A in the presence of NADPH to give 6-methylsalicylic acid, has been isolated by several groups and studied in some detail.[11] No intermediate has been found from the starting material acetyl coenzyme A to the product 6-methylsalicylic acid [2.21]. However, if the cofactor NADPH is omitted from the enzymic synthesis triacetic acid lactone [2.27] accumulates. This substance may be regarded as a derailment byproduct of the *in vitro* enzymic synthesis, and its isolation supports the idea of a stepwise addition of acetate units to a growing polyketomethylene chain (Scheme 2.10).

[2.27, triacetic acid lactone] [2.21]

Scheme 2.10. 6-Methylsalicylic acid synthetase.

Analogous observations have been made with the enzyme chalcone synthase[12] which catalyses the key reaction in flavonoid biosynthesis—the stepwise condensation of malonyl coenzyme A units with p-coumaroyl coenzyme A to give the hypothetical tri-β-ketoacyl thioester [2.28] (Scheme 2.11). The stepwise nature of this synthesis and the formation of intermediate mono- and di-ketoacyl-thioesters may similarly be deduced from the formation of enzymic derailment products [2.29]–[2.30]. These compounds are not found in the whole organism, and are by-products of the *in vitro* enzymic synthesis.

As to the question of the factor (or factors) which determine the overall pattern of cyclization of the polyketide chain, it has been suggested that the initial point of folding is the key one and that, once the first aryl ring has been produced subsequent cyclization may well proceed spontaneously—the 'zip fastener' effect. Staunton[13] has speculated that this may be initiated via the formation of a *cis*-enol or enol ether. This concept is illustrated in the Scheme 2.12 for the synthesis of physcion [2.31] an anthraquinone methyl ether found in *Polygonum* and *Rumex* sp. Formation of the intermediate enol-ether (Scheme 2.12), it is argued, determines the initial folding pattern. Once this has been determined, subsequent cyclizations follow automatically in the direction shown. As each ring is formed, appropriate sections of the polyketide are brought together and the next cyclization facilitated.

2.7 Structure determination and biomimetic synthesis

The importance of the acetate hypothesis has undoubtedly been its success in predicting the biological origins of a whole range of previously unrelated natural products and in stimulating experimental work to uncover these origins. It has also proved to be of considerable value in more chemical terms—those of structure determination and biomimetic synthesis. One of the first successful applications of the acetate hypothesis was indeed in its application[1] to the

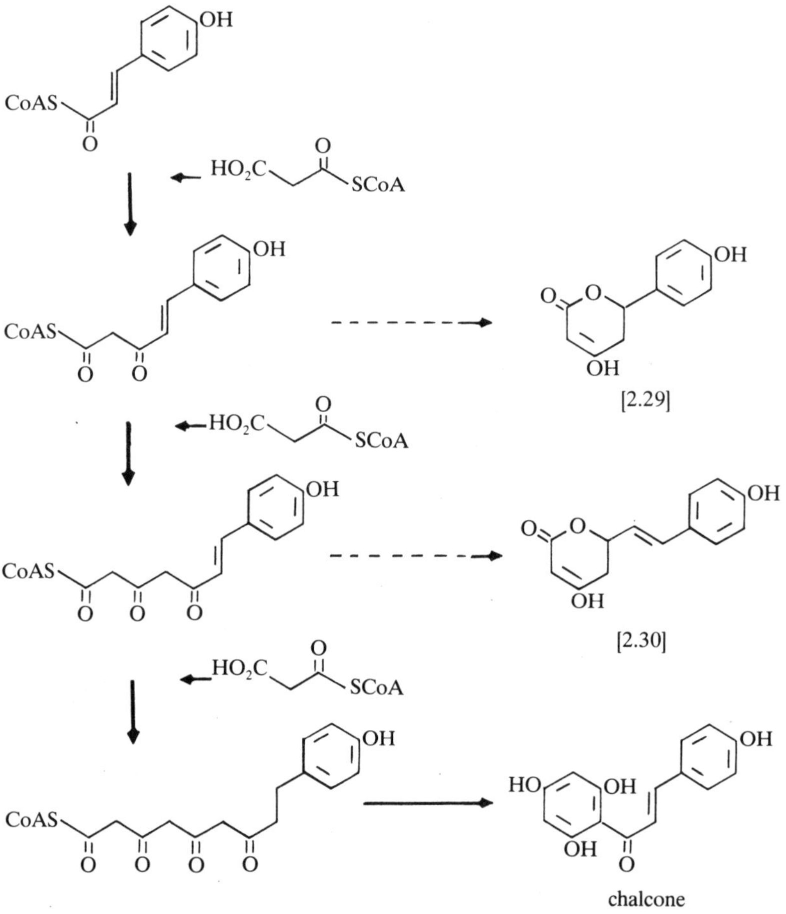

Scheme 2.11. Mechanism of action of chalcone synthase.[12]

revision of the structure of a natural product eleutherinol [2.32]. The structure [2.33] had previously been assigned to this chromone derivative on the basis of chemical work, but, as Birch indicated,[1] such a structure cannot be simply constructed from a head-to-tail linkage of acetate units. An alternative structure [2.32] was proposed, conforming to the acetate hypothesis and reappraisal of the earlier degradative evidence confirmed this structure for eleutherinol. The concept has been successfully applied in numerous other cases of natural product structure determination.[14]

The famous synthesis of tropinone announced by Robinson[15] in 1917, demonstrated the intrinsic elegance of synthetic methods based on the premise that natural substances could be synthesized in the laboratory under physiological conditions, and using components which simulated those presumed to be used in nature. It is, however, only relatively recently that these same

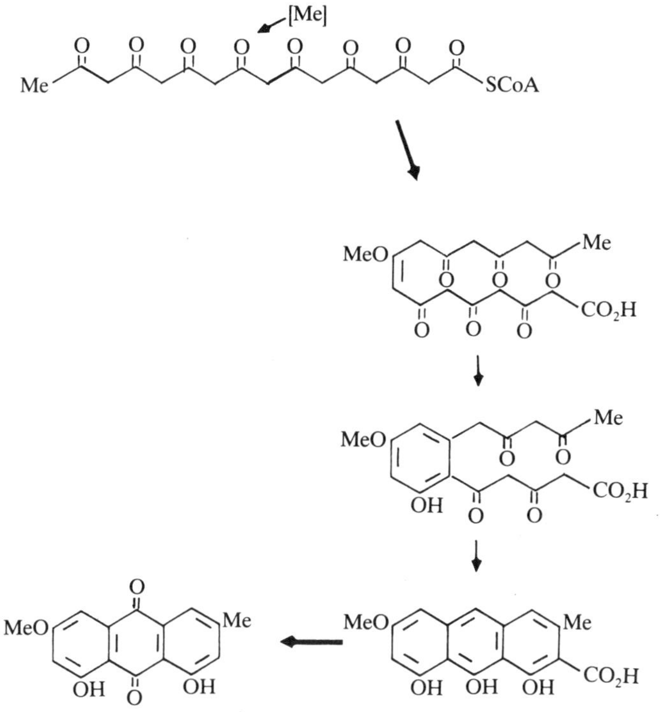

[2.31, physcion]

Scheme 2.12. Folding of the polyketide chain: biosynthesis of physcion.

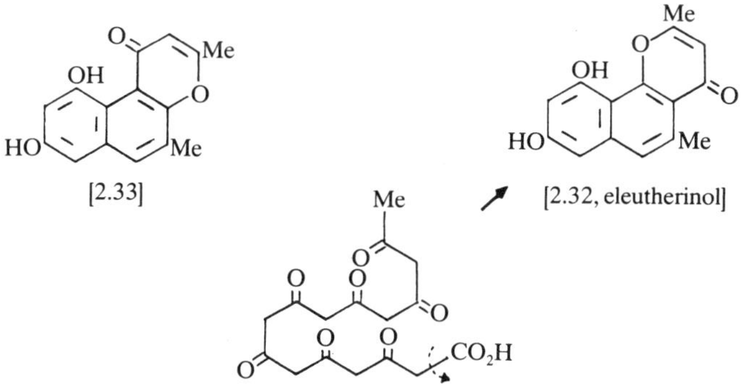

[2.33]

[2.32, eleutherinol]

ideas have begun to bear forth their promised fruit in the field of organic synthesis.[13, 16] Biomimetic syntheses may be designed on the basis of their biogenetic relevance—to test the mechanistic validity of a key step or steps in a biosynthetic pathway—or because of their synthetic utility and efficiency. It is dangerous, however, to press such laboratory analogies too far, and the ultimate success of a biogenetically-patterned synthesis does not, by itself, constitute evidence of the operation of a particular pathway *in vitro*. Nevertheless, the striking success which has attended certain biomimetic syntheses lends credence to the idea that similar enzyme catalysed processes may operate in Nature. It is on this basis that one may view many of the remarkably successful syntheses which have been described in recent years and which derive their rationale from the acetate hypothesis. In particular, they underline the facile nature of the aldol condensation reactions which occur in poly-β-ketomethylene compounds to form aromatic systems.

The early work in this field is due to Collie[2] who demonstrated that dehydroacetic acid [2.34]—a potential β-triketone [2.35]—was converted to orcinol [2.36] by base. These (and related) experimental observations led Collie to suggest that similar reactions may occur in Nature, and his statements are frequently regarded as the first tentative outline of the acetate hypothesis.

[2.34, dehydroacetic acid]

[2.35]

[2.36, orcinol]

Studies of biomimetic syntheses of polyketide metabolites have been hampered by the inaccessibility and instability of the appropriate poly-β-ketomethylene substrates. Recent work[13, 16] has, however, provided access to polycarbonyl compounds having one or more of the carbonyl groups masked, and to free poly-β-ketomethylene compounds themselves. One approach has its origins in Collie's observations and uses pyrones as masked carbonyl precursors. Another very effective approach is that adopted by Harris and his colleagues.[16] Illustrative of this method is its imaginative use[17] in the synthesis of barakol, 6-hydroxymusizin, and eleutherinol (Schemes 2.13 and 2.14).

References

1. BIRCH, A. J. *Proc. Chem. Soc.*, 3 (1962).
   BIRCH, A. J. and DONOVAN F. W. *Aust. J. Chem* 6, 360 (1953).
   RICKARDS, R. W. in *Chemistry of natural phenolic compounds* (ed. W. D. Ollis). Pergamon Press, Oxford (1961).

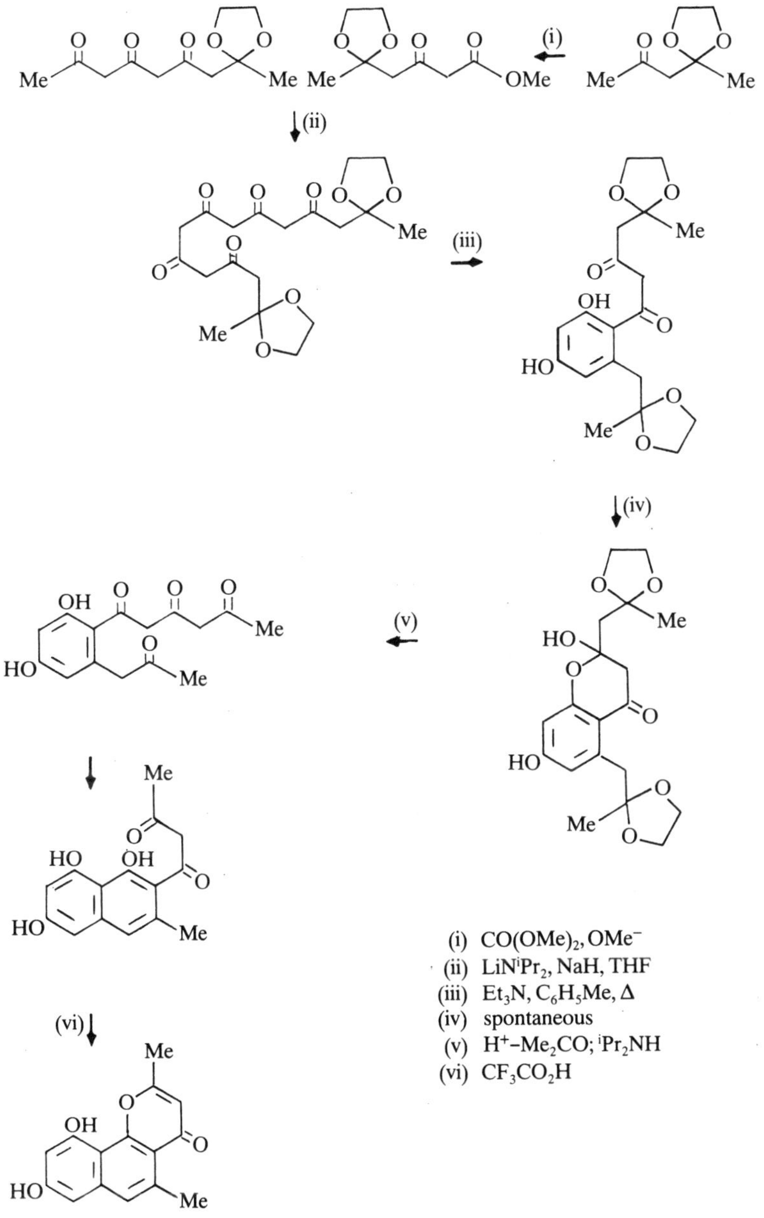

(i) $CO(OMe)_2, OMe^-$
(ii) LiN^iPr_2, NaH, THF
(iii) Et_3N, C_6H_5Me, Δ
(iv) spontaneous
(v) H^+–Me_2CO; $^iPr_2NH$
(vi) CF_3CO_2H

[2.32, eleutherinol]
Eleutherine tuberosa

Scheme 2.13. Biomimetic synthesis of eleutherinol.(17)

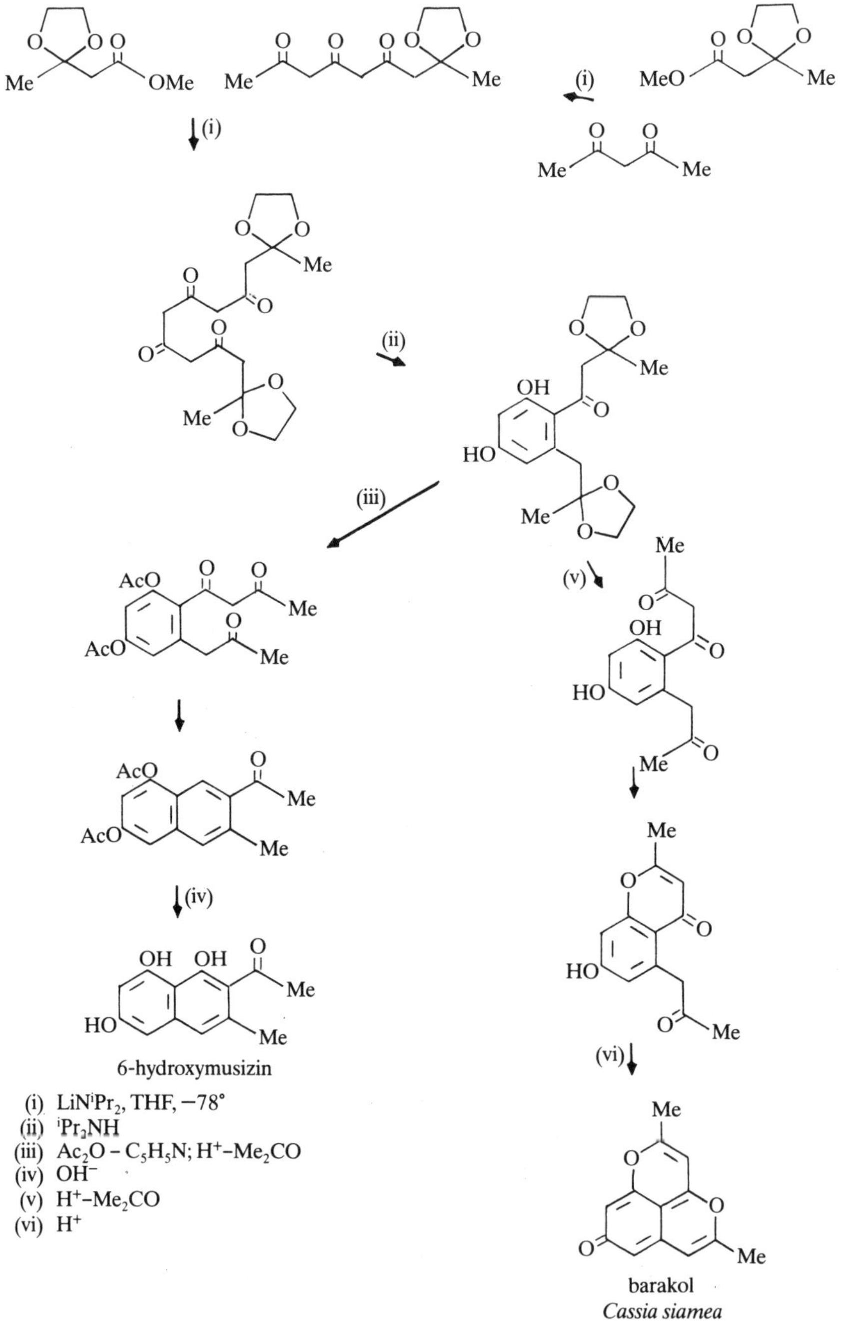

6-hydroxymusizin

(i) LiN^{i}Pr$_2$, THF, $-78°$
(ii) ^{i}Pr$_2$NH
(iii) Ac$_2$O $-$ C$_5$H$_5$N; H$^+$$-Me_2$CO
(iv) OH$^-$
(v) H$^+$$-Me_2$CO
(vi) H$^+$

barakol
Cassia siamea

Scheme 2.14. Biomimetic synthesis of 6-hydroxymusizin and barakol.[17]

2. COLLIE, J. N. *J. Chem. Soc.* **91**, 1806 (1907).
COLLIE, J. N. and MYERS, W. S., ibid. **63**, 122 (1893).

3. ROBINSON, R. *The structural relationships of natural products*. Clarendon Press, Oxford (1955).

4. HARRIS, S. M., ROBERTSON, J. S., and HARRIS, T. M. *J. Am. Chem. Soc.* **98**, 5380 (1976).

5. CANONICA, J. and SCOLASTICO, C. *J. Chem. Soc. Perkin Transactions 1*, 2639 (1972).

6. BARTON, D. H. R. and COHEN, T. *Festschrift A. Stoll*, p. 117. Birkhaüser, Basle (1957).
SCOTT, A. I., *Chem. Soc. Q. Rev.* **19**, 1 (1965).
TAYLOR, W. I. and BATTERSBY, A. R., *Oxidative coupling of phenols*. Marcel Dekker, New York (1967).

7. ZAMIR, L. O. *The biosynthesis of mycotoxins* (ed. P. S. Steyn), p. 223. Academic Press, London and New York (1980).

8. STEYN, P. S., VLEGGARR, R., and WESSELS, P. L. in *The biosynthesis of mycotoxins* (ed. P. S. Steyn), p. 105. Academic Press, London and New York (1980).

9. RINEHART, K. L. *Acc. Chem. Res.* **5**, 57 (1972).
WHITE, R. S., MARTINELLI, E., GALLO, G. G., LANSINI, G., and BENYON, P. *Nature, Lond.* **243**, 273 (1973).
JOHNSON, R. D., HABER, A., and RINEHART, K. L. *J. Am. Chem. Soc.* **96**, 3316 (1974).

10. GRISEBACH, H. and HOFHEINZ, W. *J. R. Inst. Chem.* 332–340 (1964).
GRISEBACH, H. *Biosynthetic patterns in microorganisms and plants*. John Wiley, London (1967).

11. LYNEN, F. *J. pure appl. Chem.* **14**, 137 (1967).
MURPHY, G. and LYNEN, F. *Eur. J. Biochem* **3**, 238 (1974).

12. HAHLBROCK, K. in *The biochemistry of plants*, vol. 7 (ed. E. E. Conn), p. 428. Academic Press, London and New York (1981).

13. STAUNTON, J. in *Further perspectives in organic chemistry*, Ciba Foundation Symposium 53, p. 131. Elsevier, Amsterdam and New York (1978).

14. GEISSMAN, T. A. and CROUT, D. H. G. *Organic chemistry of secondary plant metabolism*, Freeman-Cooper, San Francisco (1969).
BIRCH, A. J. in *Further perspectives in organic chemistry*, Ciba Foundation Symposium 53, p. 20. Elsevier, Amsterdam and New York (1978).

15. ROBINSON, R. *J. Chem. Soc.* **111**, 762 (1917).

16. HARRIS, T. M., HARRIS, C. M. and HINDLEY, K. B. *Progress of the chemistry of organic natural products*, vol. 31 (ed. W. Herz, H. Grisebach, and G. W. Kirby), p. 217. Springer-Verlag, Vienna (1973).
MONEY, T. *Chem. Rev.* **70**, 553 (1970).

17. HARRIS, T. M. and WITTEK, P. J. *J. Am. Chem. Soc.* **97**, 3270 (1975).

3

ALKALOIDS AND NITROGEN-CONTAINING AMINO-ACID METABOLITES

3.1 Introduction

Although only some 10–15 per cent of vascular plants and some fungi metabolize alkaloids studies of their chemistry exercised a profound influence upon organic chemistry as it evolved. Some alkaloids are quite toxic (for example the fatal dose of nicotine in man is 40 mg; that for strychnine rather less); others when administered to mammals give rise to significant physiological responses. For these reasons, therefore, much of the chemistry of alkaloids has been intimately associated with medicine and the development of potential therapeutic agents. Speculations on the biogenetic origins of alkaloids likewise occupy an important niche in the evolution of biogenetic thought. Many of the early ideas on biogenesis originated from the specific problems posed by alkaloids, but there is little doubt that their great overall contribution was correctly to orientate biogentic thinking in terms of chemical mechanisms and biochemical compatability.[1]

Structurally, alkaloids represent a very diverse and heterogeneous group of compounds.[2] They are characterized by the presence of one or more nitrogen atoms which, as their name indicates, frequently but not invariably have a basic nature. Because of their general complexity, the nomenclature of alkaloids has not been effectively systematized. Usually it is accomplished on the basis of the plant source and the general similarity of molecular structure. The nitrogen atom(s) may be present in an acyclic system, (these substances are often referred to as protoalkaloids), but frequently forms part of a heterocyclic ring. Some examples of the range of ring systems and the bewildering diversity of structural types found amongst the alkaloids are shown in Fig. 3.1. Paradoxically, it was this structural complexity which gave the major impetus to the elaboration of biogenetic theories; the wish and the belief of chemists to sketch in the underlying biological themes and so bring some order and rationale to alkaloids and alkaloid chemistry.

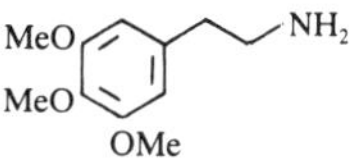

mescalin [tyrosine]

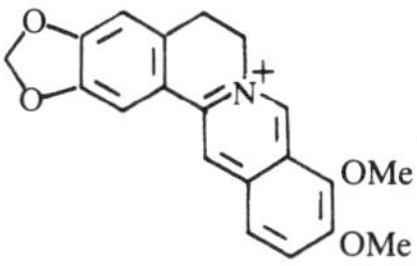

berberine [tyrosine]

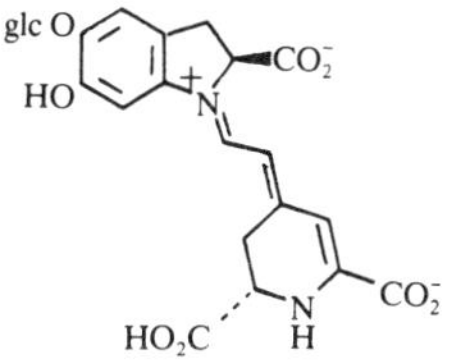

betanidin [tyrosine]

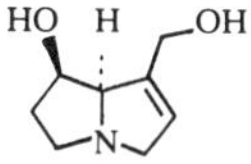

retronecine [ornithine]

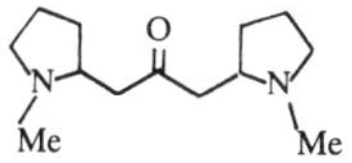

cuscohygrine [ornithine, acetic acid]

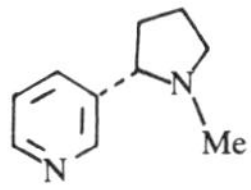

nicotine [ornithine, nicotinic acid]

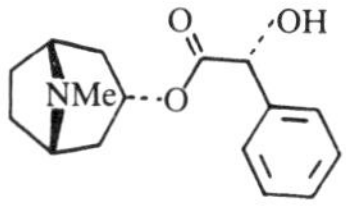

hyoscyamine
[ornithine, phenylalanine]

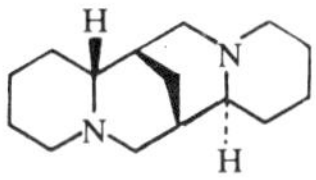

sparteine [lysine]

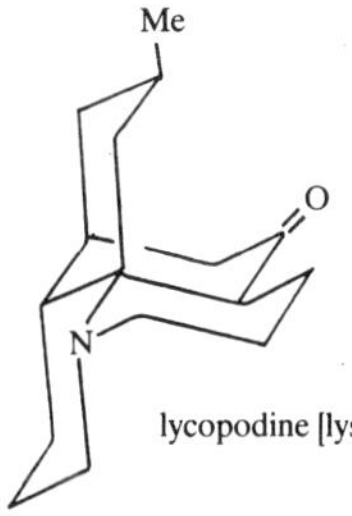

lycopodine [lysine, acetic acid]

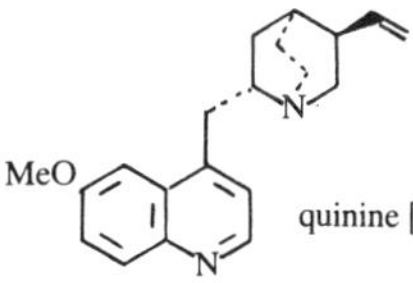

quinine [tryptophan, mevalonic acid]

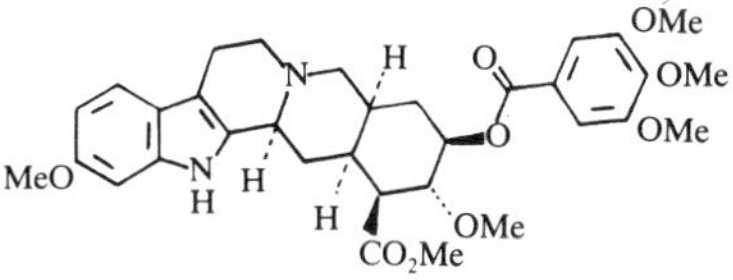

reserpine [tryptophan, mevalonic acid]

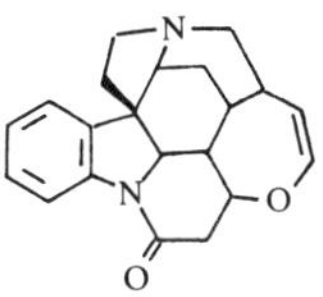

strychnine [tryptophan, mevalonic and acetic acids]

Fig. 3.1. Some alkaloids and their biosynthetic precursors.

3.2 Early ideas

As early as 1910 Winterstein and Trier[2] in a remarkably percipient book, suggested that the α-amino-acids ornithine [3.1], lysine [3.2], phenylalanine [3.3], and tryptophan [3.5], might serve as the starting points for the phytochemical synthesis of alkaloids. Seven years later, Robinson's ambitious yet convincing formulation of biogenetic schemes[3] to the alkaloids, highlighted for the first time the importance to natural products chemistry of biogenetic theory and firmly established the right intellectual climate for such studies. Retrospectively, it may be seen that, apart from the general framework of ideas which he set up, two striking observations ensured the success of Robinson's theories. The first was his tropinone synthesis, the second his conception of the relationship between the morphine—thebaine group of alkaloids and the then well-known benzyl-isoquinoline system. 'Such ideas come to few men.'

Robinson's synthesis of tropinone[4] was simple and direct and contrasted sharply with the classical synthesis of the same base announced earlier by Willstätter. The synthesis is perhaps not properly described as biomimetic, although it is analogous in several important respects to the biosynthetic route now known to be adopted in Nature to the tropane skeleton, as in hyoscyamine[5] (Fig. 3.2). With few exceptions, alkaloids of this class are found only in species of certain genera of the plant family Solanaceae. The pathway illustrated to hyoscyamine was deduced on the basis of various isotopic tracer experiments which establish the identity of intermediates and their sequence on the path. An interesting facet of this route is the unsymmetrical incorporation of ornithine into the tropane skeleton. Pathways to other alkaloids in which ornithine (and the related amino acid, lysine) are involved display a similar specificity, whilst for others it must be concluded that the biosynthetic pathway leads through a symmetrical four (or five) carbon intermediate, (*vide infra*).

The second observation which underpinned the success of Robinson's ideas was his suggestion, based on biogenetic arguments, of the relationship of the morphine–thebaine alkaloids to those of the more familiar benzyl-isoquinoline bases.[1] The crucial step in the process of reasoning was that if the benzyl-isoquinoline ring system were folded in a particular manner then formation of a new carbon–carbon bond gave the morphine skeleton (Fig. 3.3).

Few can fail to be moved by the beauty and simplicity of Robinson's idea, and by the subsequent experimental work of Battersby[6] and Barton,[7] which demonstrated the detailed pathway between norlaudanosoline [3.6] and morphine [3.7] (Scheme 3.1). In passing, one may note once again in this scheme the importance of oxidative phenol coupling[8] in the formation of a secondary metabolite, and the manner in which selective O-methylation orients the substrate to a particular mode of oxidative coupling. The final O-demethylation step to give morphine itself should also be noted.

Robinson's tropinone synthesis (1917)

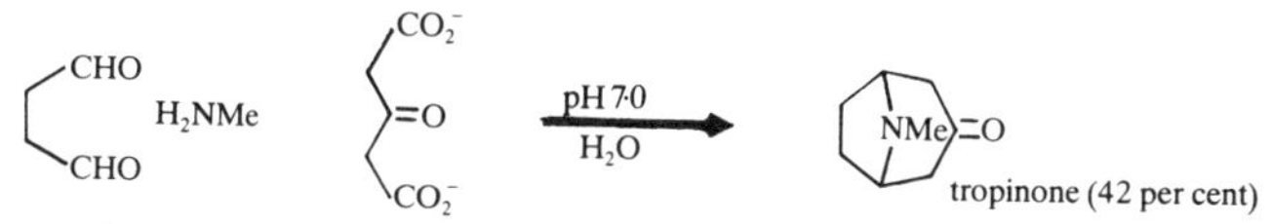

Biosynthesis of hyoscyamine (after Leete[5])

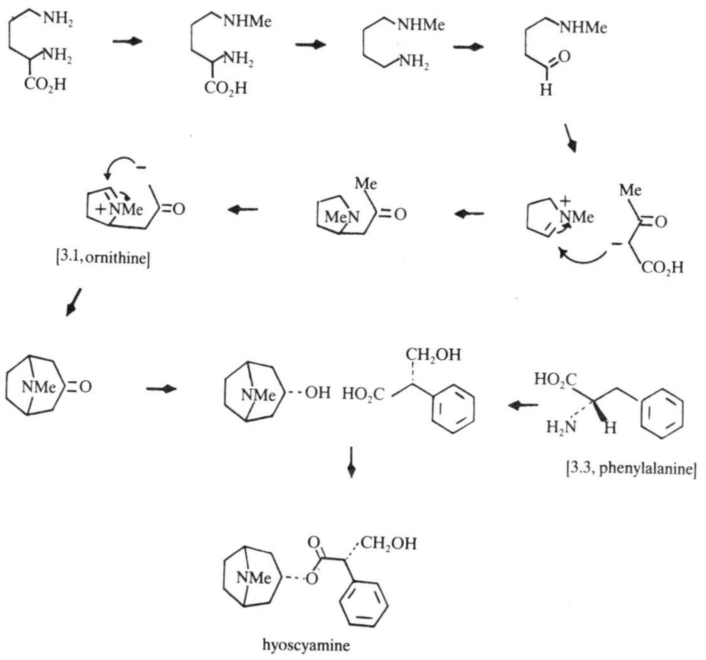

Fig. 3.2.

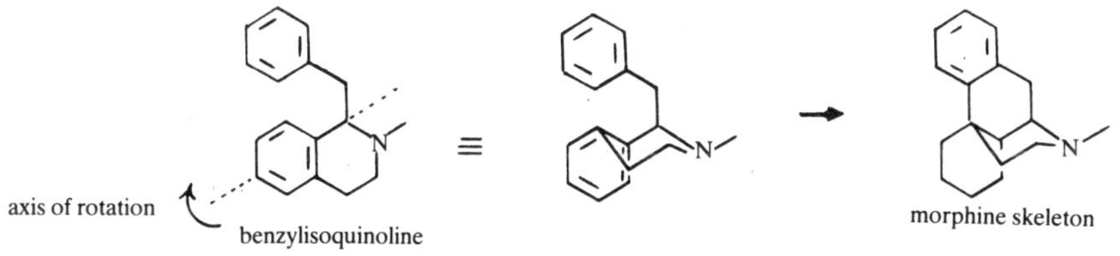

Fig. 3.3. The morphine skeleton.

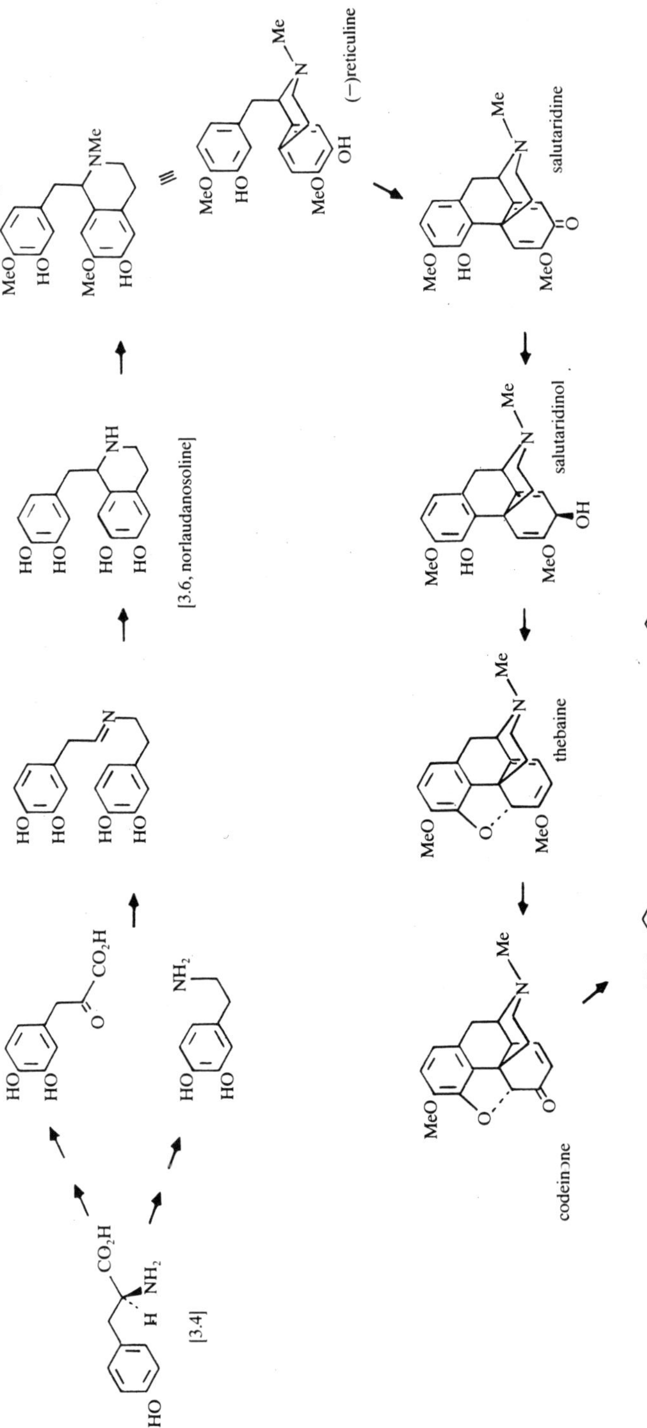

Scheme 3.1. Biosynthesis of morphine.(7,8)

3.3 Biogenetic theories of alkaloid metabolism

The cornerstones of Robinson's theories, and those of later workers, were the recognition of structural relationships and the firm assertion that Nature employs recognizable chemical processes.[1] Thus, it was observed that the structures of many alkaloids could be dissected into fragments whose C–N skeleton bore a close correspondence to one or other of a small group of amino-acids [3.1]–[3.4]. It was further argued that their *in vivo* assembly into alkaloids should be explicable in terms of rational chemical mechanisms. In addition to the reactions encountered in acetate metabolism (carbanion condensations, O- and C-alkylation, decarboxylation and oxidation and reduction), certain additional types of process were postulated to be of major importance in alkaloid biosynthesis— Schiff's base formation (i), the Mannich condensation in its several guises (ii), and various oxidation or dehydrogenation reactions (iii). If to these one adds some of the known *in vivo* transformations of α-amino-acids[9] (Scheme 3.2), then one has the rough complement of chemical reactions involved in alkaloid biosynthesis.

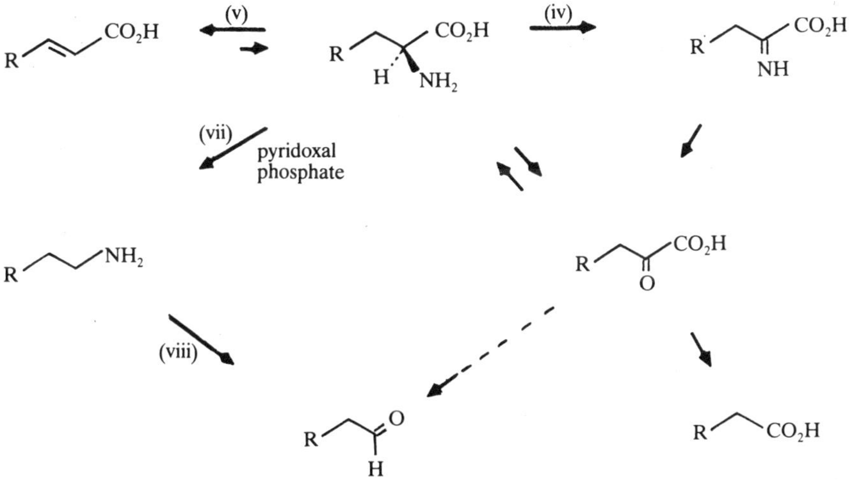

Scheme 3.2. Metabolism of α-amino-acids.[9]

When available in excess of cellular requirements, most nitrogen compounds, including α-amino-acids, may be utilized by the organism in alternative ways. Their overall levels in the cell are balanced by synthesis, degradation and other transformations. In Scheme 3.2 are shown some of the more common ways in which α-amino-acids are metabolized by deamination, transamination, and decarboxylation. Amino-acid oxidases are typical FAD oxidative deaminases, and catalyse the conversion of the α-amino-acid to the α-keto-acid via the corresponding imine (iv). For some amino acids, such as phenylalanine, loss of ammonia to give the unsaturated acid is another important mode of deamination (v). Transamination (vi) provides for amino-nitrogen transfer and involves the reversible transfer of the amino-group from the α-amino-acid to an α-keto-acid. The transamination step is often the first one in the dedgradation of most α-amino-acids. A further important general reaction of α-amino-acids is their de-carboxylation to amines (vii), for which pyridoxal phosphate is a cofactor. Finally, mono- and di-amine-oxidases, which utilize FAD as coenzymes, are responsible for the conversion of primary amines to the corresponding aldehydes (viii).

The association of these various reaction types (i)—(viii) with the amino-acid ornithine [3.1] in the proposed pathway of biosynthesis of the alkaloid hyo-scyamine are shown in Fig. 3.2. The status of ornithine (as the ultimate pre-cursor) and N-methylputrescine (as an intermediate) has been demonstrated by tracer studies, and these are then linked to the final product by a series of mechanistically plausible steps.

The basis of biogenetic thinking about alkaloids was and still is the recogni-tion of common structural patterns which can be related to a handful of α-amino-acids—ornithine [3.1], lysine [3.2], phenylalanine [3.3], tyrosine [3.4], and tryptophan [3.5]. To these one may also now add nicotinic acid [3.8] and anthranilic acid [3.9]. These lines of thought are illustrated below for three groups of alkaloids and interpreted in terms of more recent experimental work.

[3.1, $n = 3$, ornithine]
[3.2, $n = 4$, lysine]

[3.3, R = H, phenylalanine]
[3.4, R = OH, tyrosine]

[3.5, tryptophan]

[3.8, nicotinic acid]

[3.9, anthranilic acid]

3.4 Alkaloids based on ornithine and lysine

Part of the folklore of biogenetic theory concerns the early observations made by Robinson[1] on the alkaloids derived from ornithine (the pyrolidine group) and those from lysine (the piperidine group). This work was based on the identification of the C_4-N unit (derived from ornithine) and the C_5-N unit (derived from lysine) as structural entities in these alkaloids. These are shown (in heavy print) in two groups of alkaloids (Fig. 3.4). As these examples show there is some degree of resemblance between the two groups and they may be regarded, at least in outline, as homologous. Key intermediates in the biosynthesis of these

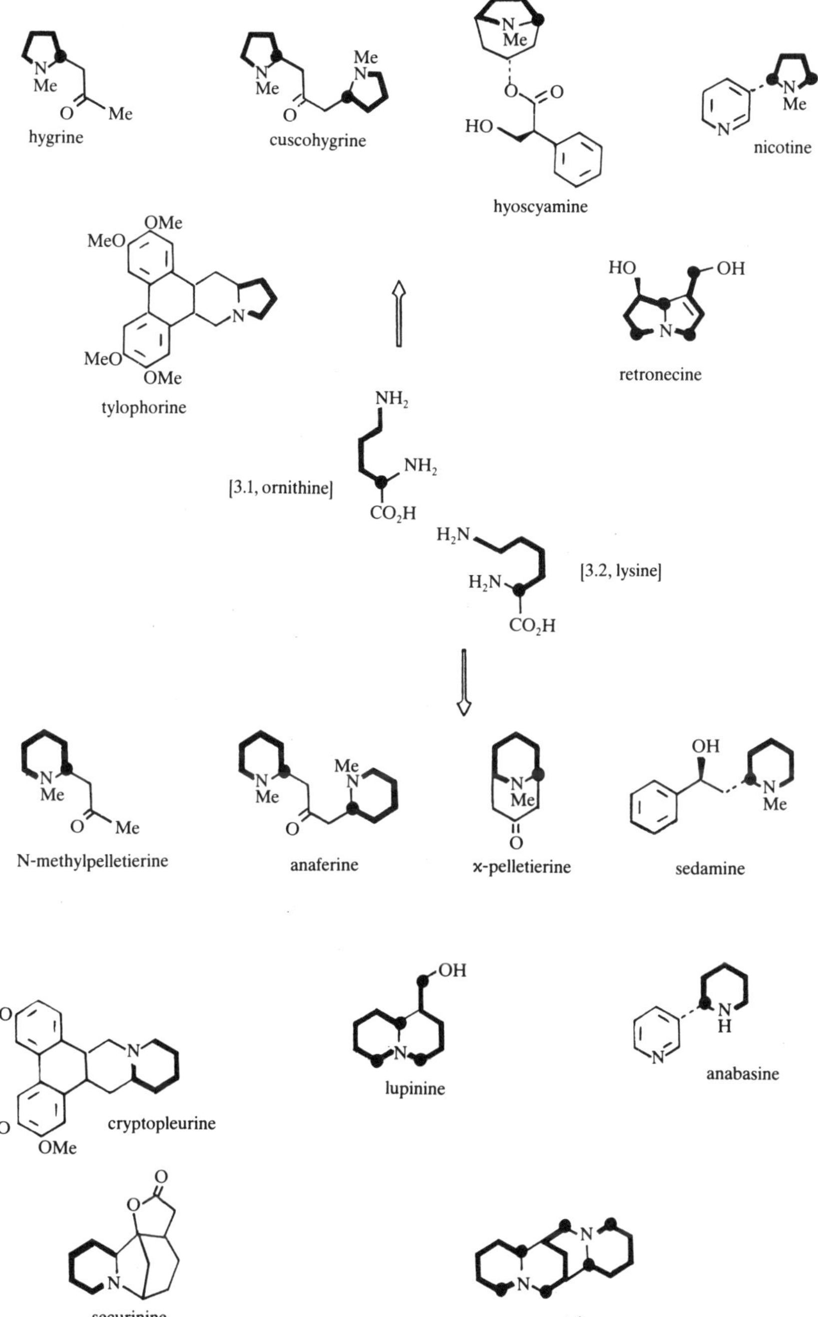

Fig. 3.4. Alkaloids derived biosynthetically from ornithine and lysine.

alkaloids are the acyclic amino-aldehydes and the cyclic Shiff's bases with which they are in equilibrium.

A fascinating aspect of the experimental biosynthetic work on these alkaloids concerns the 'symmetrical' or 'non-symmetrical' incorporation of the amino-acid skeleton (minus the carboxyl group) into the alkaloid structures.[10] This facet of metabolism is illustrated by the positions of incorporation of ^{14}C isotopic label ($\bullet$) in the alkaloid metabolites derived respectively from 2-^{14}C—ornithine and lysine (Fig. 3.4). Thus assimilation of ornithine into the C_4-N unit of hygrine, cuscohygrine, and hyoscyamine is asymmetric; that is, C-2 and C-5 of the amino-acid skeleton retain their identity. This contrasts with nicotine and retronecine where C-2 and C-5 assume equivalence in the final alkaloid. Analogously, the C_5-N unit derived from lysine is incorporated into anabasine, sedamine, N-methylputrescine, anaferine, and halosaline in an asymmetric manner. Whereas in the alkaloids, lupinine and sparteine C-2 and C-6 do not preserve their individual identity and a symmetrical C_5-N unit appears to be incorporated. This apparent paradox posed by the results of various tracer experiments[10] was most elegantly and ingeniously resolved by Spenser and Leistner.[11] Some of the crucial tracer experiments which influenced the development of their hypothesis are shown in Fig. 3.5. It was deduced from these experiments that a symmetrical compound such as the diamine cadaverine [3.10] could not be an intermediate between lysine [3.2] and the alkaloids anabasine and sedamine. Yet it was also clear that isotopic label was incorporated, non-randomly, into anabasine [3.11] from 1,5-^{14}C$_2$ cadaverine [3.10], Fig. 3.6, and in order to explain this apparent anomaly it was considered that the utilization of cadaverine in piperidine alkaloid biosynthesis was an aberrant process. Spenser and Leistner's theory[11] gratifyingly accommodates each of these findings.

The model is outlined in Scheme 3.3. It assumes that initially L-lysine [3.2] undergoes stereospecific decarboxylation *via* its pyridoxal phosphate adduct and L-lysine decarboxylase. The product of this reaction is a cadaverine-pyridoxal adduct [3.12] and in the second stage this undergoes stereospecific oxidative deamination to yield 5-aminopentanal or its internal Schiff's base Δ^1-piperideine [3.13] the immediate precursor of the various piperidine alkaloids. A pathway of this type fully explains the asymmetric incorporation of L-lysine [3.2] into the piperidine ring with retention of the C-2 hydrogen. It is assumed that in this instance the equilibrium constant between the free and bound cadaverine [3.10] $\rightleftharpoons$ [3.12] strongly favours the bound form [3.12]. The model accounts not only for the assimilation of cadaverine and the asymmetric incorporation of L-lysine, but also for the origin of those piperidine alkaloids into which a lysine-derived C_5-N unit is incorporated in a symmetrical fashion (Fig. 3.4). If the equilibrium constant controlling the dissociation of bound cadaverine favours free cadaverine [3.10], then symmetrical incorporation is assured. Presumably, the same model may be employed to rationalize the analogous observations made with the amino-acid L-ornithine [3.1] and the pyrrolidine alkaloids (Fig. 3.4).

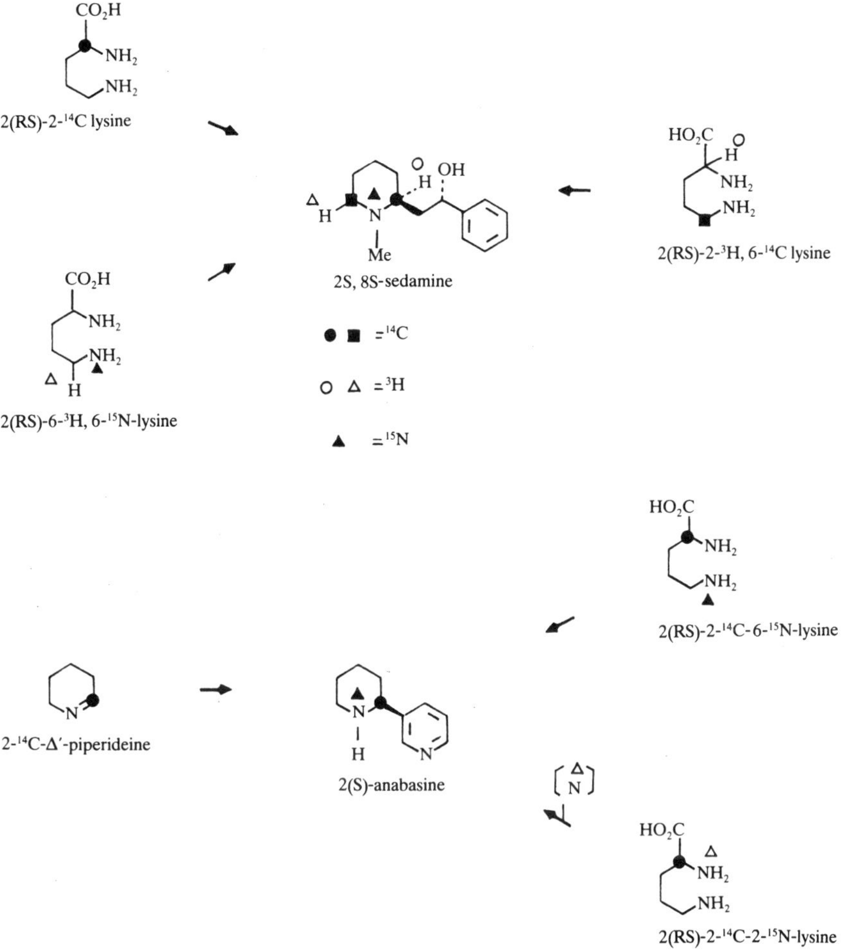

Fig. 3.5. Tracer experiments with piperidine alkaloids.[11]

Fig. 3.6. Incorporation of cadaverine into anabasine.

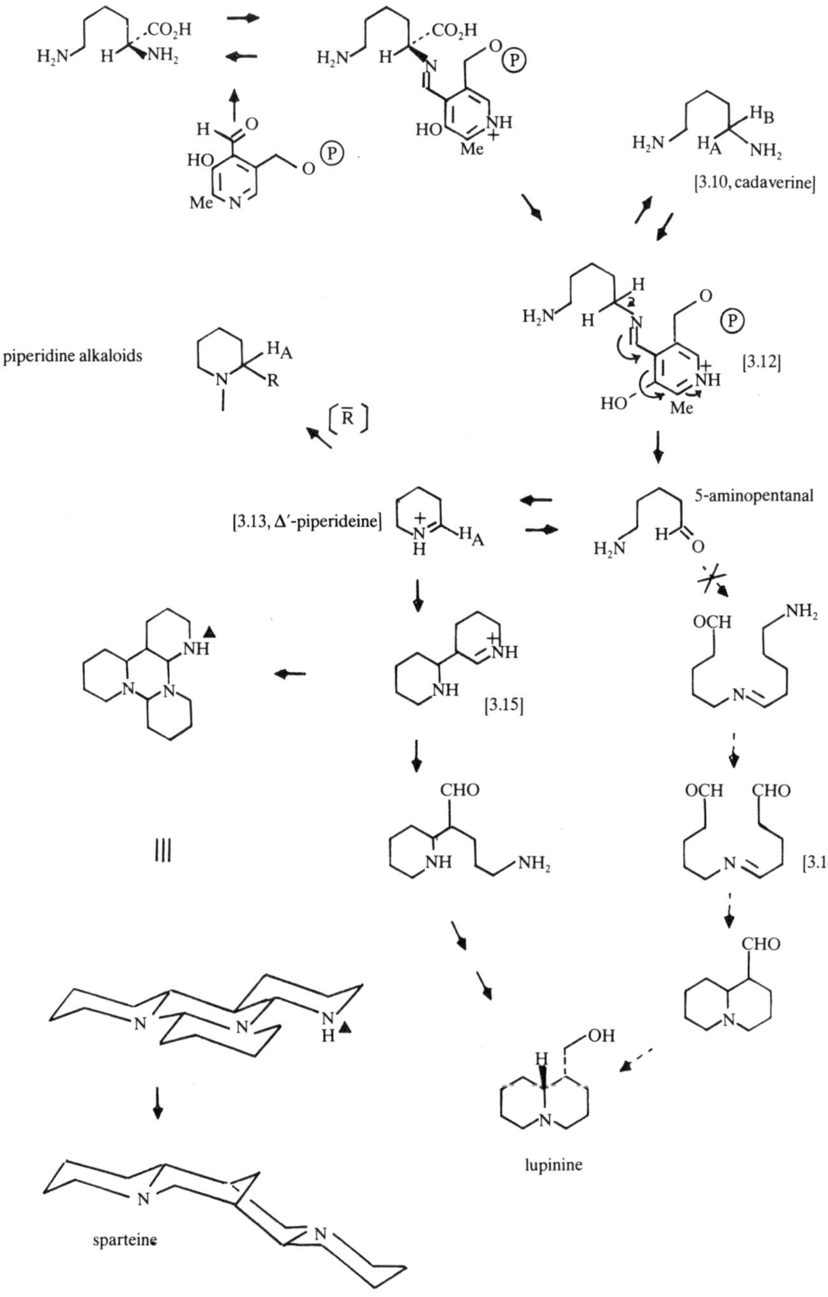

Scheme 3.3. Biosynthesis of piperidine alkaloids from L-lysine.[11]

The carbon skeleton of lupinine (Fig. 3.4, Scheme 3.3) the major alkaloid of *Lupinus luteus* is derived from *two* C_5-N units related to lysine. The distribution of isotopic tracer, incorporated from either DL-lysine or its decarboxylation product cadaverine [3.10], in the alkaloid was consistent with the intermediacy on the biosynthetic pathway of the symmetrical dialdehyde ([3.14] route A) or the dissymmetric Δ^1-piperideine dimer ([3.15] route B). A ^{13}C, ^{15}N tracer study has confirmed[11] that the alkaloid is generated *in vivo* from two cadaverine units and by a route (e.g. route B) which excludes intermediates such as [3.14] with C_{2V} symmetry.

Likewise, sparteine (Fig. 3.1, Scheme 3.3), which occurs in a number of stereoisomeric forms, is biosynthesized from *three* cadaverine derived C_5-N units by a pathway which again excludes intermediates with C_{2V} symmetry. Here, Spenser and his collaborators[11] favour a pathway which encompasses the rearrangement of isotripiperidine—a trimeric form of Δ^1-piperideine [3.13]—followed by elimination of one nitrogen atom (▲ either oxidatively or by displacement, Scheme 3.3)—an interesting mechanistic puzzle!

3.4.1 Biosynthesis of pyrrolizidine alkaloids

Pyrrolizidine alkaloids have a wide distribution and are particularly characteristic of genera of the plant families Compositae, Leguminosae, and Boraginaceae. The fused bicyclic ring system characteristic of these alkaloids is derived from the amino-acid L-ornithine [3.1] via the diamine putrescine [3.18] and the symmetrical dialdehyde (C_4-N-C_4) intermediate [3.19]. A plausible scheme of biogenesis for the alkaloid trachelanthamidine [3.20] was outlined (Scheme 3.4, →) on this basis by Geissman and Crout.[12]

Retronecine [3.16] is the most commonly found basic portion of the pyrrolizidine alkaloids (e.g. retrorsine [3.17]) and much of the *in vivo* biosynthetic work has concentrated on this base. In accord with the pathway of biogenesis (Scheme 3.4), putrescine [3.18] is incorporated with high efficiency (up to 5.2 per cent) into retronecine [3.16], such that the use of ^{13}C as an isotopic tracer is permitted (Fig. 3.7). *Senecio isatideus* plants fed 1,4-^{13}C$_2$-putrescine [3.18*a*] gave retronecine which showed enhanced signals for C-3, 5, 8 and 9. Similarly, 2,3-^{13}C$_2$-putrescine [3.18*b*] gave analogous enhancement of the two pairs of doublets corresponding to C-1/C-2 and C-6/C-7 in the ^{13}C n.m.r. spectrum of retronecine. Later work by Kahn and Robins[13] identified the immediate precursor of the dialdehyde [3.19] in the biosynthetic sequence as N-(4-aminobutyl)-1,4-diaminobutane (homospermidine [3.21]). This latter base, labelled with ^{14}C, was also efficiently transformed to retronecine [3.16] *in vivo*. Homospermidine was also demonstrated to be a natural constituent of *S. isatideus* plants and its acceptance as a true biosynthetic intermediate necessitates a modification of the suggested pathway of Geissman and Crout[12] (Scheme 3.4 →). It is interesting to note in passing, that the evidence in this

instance points to the intermediary of a C_8-N symmetrical dialdehyde intermediate [3.19]. This contrasts with the case of lupinine (Scheme 3.3), where
the corresponding C_{10}-N dialdehyde [3.14] is not thought to be directly involved
in alkaloid biosynthesis.

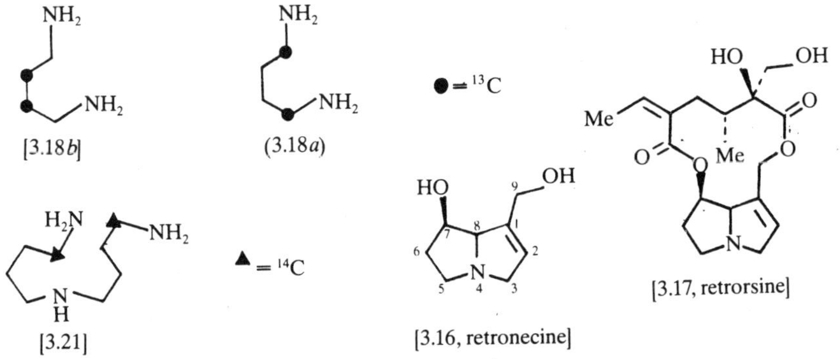

Fig. 3.7. Biosynthesis of retronecine: tracer experiments.[13]

The feasibility of this proposed biosynthetic pathway from homospermidine
[3.21] was convincingly demonstrated by Robins[13] in a biogenetically-patterned
synthesis of (±)-trachelanthamidine [3.20], carried out under physiological
conditions of pH and temperature. The triamine [3.21] was incubated with pea
seedling diamine oxidase at pH 7.0. The presumed intermediates of this reaction
[3.22] were reduced directly with sodium borohydride at 0° to give (±)-
trachelanthamidine (40 per cent). The alkaloid [3.20] was also biomimetically
synthesized from homospermidine [3.21] by a 'one pot' procedure. The substrate [3.21] was incubated with diamine oxidase and catalase at 27°, pH 7.5
then treated with liver alcohol dehydrogenase, NADH and ethanol (as hydride
donor) to give (±)-trachelanthamidine (22 per cent).

3.5 Alkaloids based on the aromatic amino-acids

A noteworthy feature of secondary metabolism is the formation of a whole
spectrum of secondary metabolites by different chemical embellishment of one
key intermediate. Nowhere is this principle more eloquently illustrated than in
the various groups of alkaloids derived from the aromatic amino-acids—L-
phenylalanine [3.3], L-tryosine [3.4], and L-tryptophan [3.5]. As the subject
moves into a new phase of development questions which are frequently posed
are . . . 'What are the purposes of this prolific synthetic activity and what is the
relationship between production, structure, and function?' Invariably, or almost
invariably, no clear answer can yet be given. Often one can only simply ponder,
depending on one's viewpoint, Nature's impressive economy, or alternatively her
unrestrained prodigality, in the biosynthetic pathways of secondary metabolism.

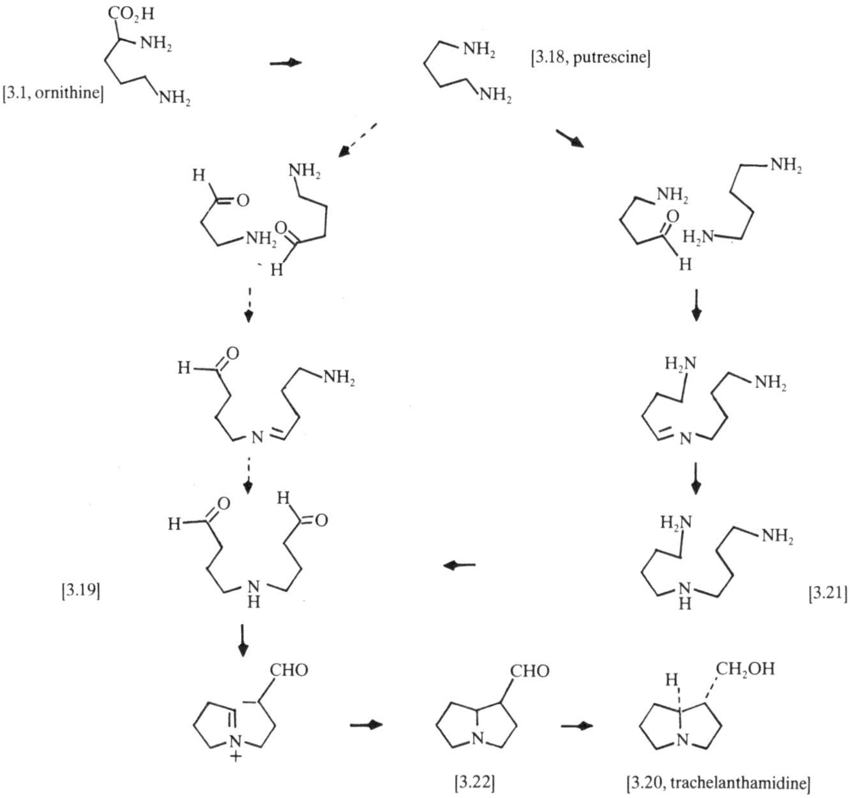

[3.1, ornithine] [3.18, putrescine]

[3.19] [3.21]

[3.22] [3.20, trachelanthamidine]

Scheme 3.4. Biosynthesis of pyrrolizidine alkaloids.[12, 13]

3.5.1 Phenylethylamine and related alkaloids

A phenylethylamine fragment is present in many alkaloids,[14] and biogenetic theories have been remarkably successful in predicting the events which lead to this group of natural products. An early postulate was that this structural unit originated from the amino-acids phenylalanine [3.3] and/or tyrosine [3.4]. Thus, Winterstein and Trier[2] suggested that the nucleus of laudanosine [3.23] was formed by condensation of dopamine [3.25] and 3,4-dihydroxyphenylacetaldehyde [3.26], and the concept was later refined and extended by Robinson, who delineated the relationship between the benzyl-tetrahydroisoquinoline skeleton and the structures of various other groups of alkaloids including those of the morphine group.[1,3] All the recent isotopic tracer work has served to underline the correctness of these views; all the structural variants (Fig. 3.8) are thus derived in principle by different transformations of one key intermediate, the benzyl-tetrahydroisoquinoline–norlaudanosoline [3.27]; although the actual process by which norlaudanosoline itself is derived has been a subject of further

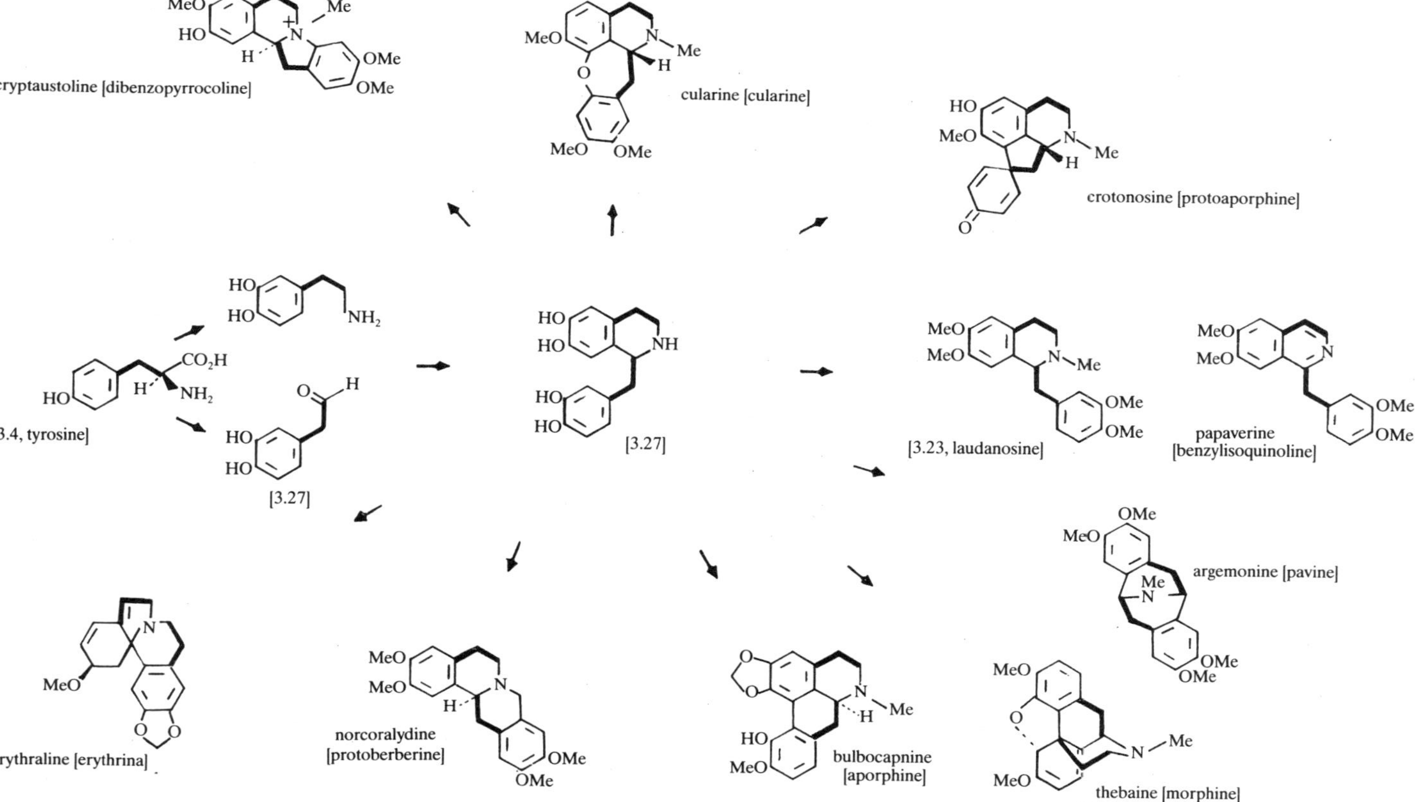

Fig. 3.8. Structured variants of the benzyl-isoquinoline carbon-nitrogen skeleton.

debate. Recent work at the enzymological level, however, favours the original concept of Winterstein and Trier,[2] in contrast to some experimental evidence that dihydroxyphenylpyruvic acid provided the benzylic unit of the intermediate [3.27].

Many plants which metabolize alkaloids from the intermediate [3.27] synthesize compounds which belong to one or more of the various skeletal types. The enzymology leading to these products is almost totally unexplored and, at the moment, speculation about the factors which direct norlaudanosoline [3.27] into one or more of the competing biosynthetic outlets is based largely on chemical reasoning. Two features appear to be important, although in themselves they do not comprise the basis of a unified hypothesis.[10] The influence of stereochemistry is highlighted by the alternative biosynthetic roles of (R) and (S)-reticuline [3.28a] and [3.28b] (Scheme 3.5). The pathway to the morphine alkaloids directly utilizes the (R) steroisomer [3.28a] whereas the (S)-(+)reticuline [3.28b] is assimilated into the berberine bridge alkaloids. An interesting facet, however, of the work in *Papaver somniferum* was the observed incorporation of both the (R) and (S) forms of reticuline [3.28a, b] into the morphine alkaloids. In order to accomodate these results, Battersby postulated[6] the presence of a 'red-ox' system in the poppy, which establishes an equilibrium between the (R) and (S) stereoisomers [3.28a, b] via the 1,2-dehydro form [3.29]. Battersby extrapolated[6] this observation to suggest that the dehydro-intermediate [3.29] might well lie at a branching point of biosynthetic pathways. In *Papaver somniferum*, the major pathway leads *via* the (R) steroisomer of reticuline [3.28a] to the morphine alkaloids; the minor pathway *via* (S)-reticuline [3.28b] to laudanosine [3.23].

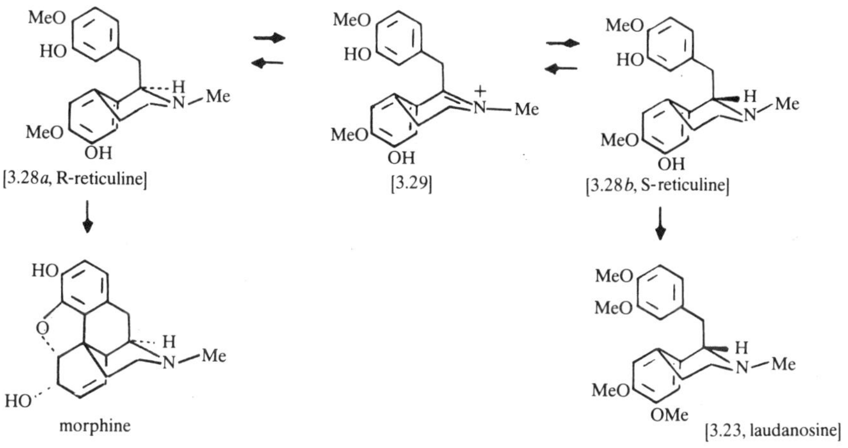

Scheme 3.5. Biosynthesis of alkaloids in *Papaver somniferum*.[6]

The significance of the O-methylation pattern of the benzyl-tetrahydroiso-quinoline precursor has been pointed out by several workers,[10] and is under-lined by the failure to incorporate isotopic label into alkaloids from putative precursors with the 'wrong' methylation pattern. Three partially-methylated derivatives of norlaudanosoline are key intermediates to the various benzyl-isoquinoline alkaloids and their derivatives—norprotosinomenine [3.30], orientaline [3.36], and reticuline [3.28]. (S)-Norprotosinomenine [3.30] leads to the erythrina group of alkaloids,[15] e.g. erythraline [3.31] and β-erythoidine [3.32] (Scheme 3.6), by an initial intramolecular para-para oxidative phenolic coupling, followed by molecular rearrangement. Norprotosinomenine [3.30] is also the immediate precursor[16] of the aporphine alkaloids—corydine [3.33], glaucine [3.34], and dicentrine [3.35] in *Dicentra exima*. Conversion occurs once more *via* oxidative coupling of the two phenolic nuclei and rearrangement.

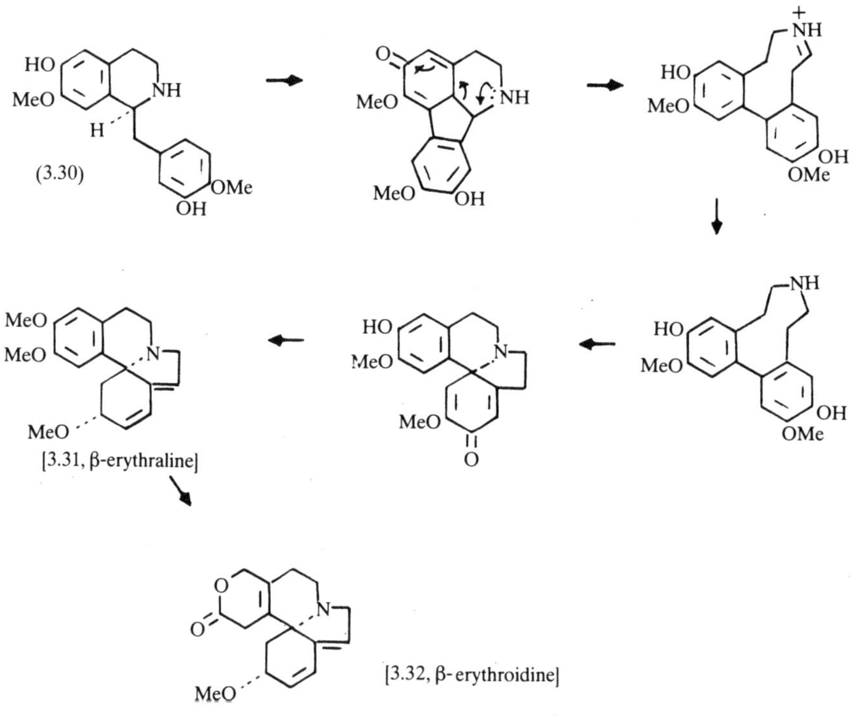

Scheme 3.6. Biosynthesis of the erythrina alkaloids.

Finally, in the opium poppy *Papaver somniferum*, orientaline [3.36] is trans-formed[17] to the aporphine alkaloid isothebaine [3.37], whereas its structural isomer (R)-reticuline [3.28a], differing only in the position of a methyl ether group, is converted to the morphine alkaloids thebaine, codeine, and morphine (Scheme 3.1).

[3.33, corydine]   [3.34, glaucine]   [3.35, dicentrine]

These and observations of a similar genre support the hypothesis that the process of O-methylation (via S-adenosyl-methionine, SAM) is a means to direct and channel oxidative cyclization along a particular pathway. The methyl ether group may be visualized in these circumstances as a form of protecting group which inactivates particular phenolic hydroxyl groups towards oxidation.

[3.36, orientaline]   [3.37, isothebaine]

Analogous observations have been made[18] with the isoquinoline alkaloids of the Amaryllidaceae (Scheme 3.7), where the methylation pattern of the precursor norbelladine [3.38] controls its entry into the biosynthetic pathways leading to the lycorine series (e.g. [3.39] initial o-p' phenolic coupling followed by cyclization onto nitrogen), to the crinine series ([3.40], p-p' coupling followed by cyclization onto nitrogen), and finally the galanthamine series. Here, phenolic coupling (p-o') occurs, but N-methylation of the norbelladine precursor blocks cyclization onto nitrogen and directs the intermediate [3.41] into the dibenzofuran pathway (e.g. [3.42]). These observations underline once again how remarkably fruitful and clairvoyant some of the earlier chemical and biogenetic predictions turn out to be. In 1957, Barton and Cohen suggested[8] that the diverse skeletal structures found among the Amaryllidaceae alkaloids were formed along the pathways indicated. Significantly, the proposals were made at a time when the occurrence of the intermediate norbelladine [3.38] had not been proven. Norbelladine [3.38] itself is now known to be formed by condensation of a tyramine (C_6C_2N) unit with a $C_6.C_1$ fragment derived from phenylalanine *via* cinnamic acid (Scheme 3.7).

The norlaudanosoline alkaloids fall into two major sub-groups. The first of these contains the erythrina, aporphine, and morphine bases (*vide supra*), based upon a $C_{16}N$ skeleton. The inclusion of an additional carbon atom into the benzyl-tetrahydroisoquinoline structure gives the skeleton of the second sub-group—the protoberberine, protopine, and benzophenanthridine bases. This additional carbon atom—the so-called 'berberine bridge'—is produced[19] by

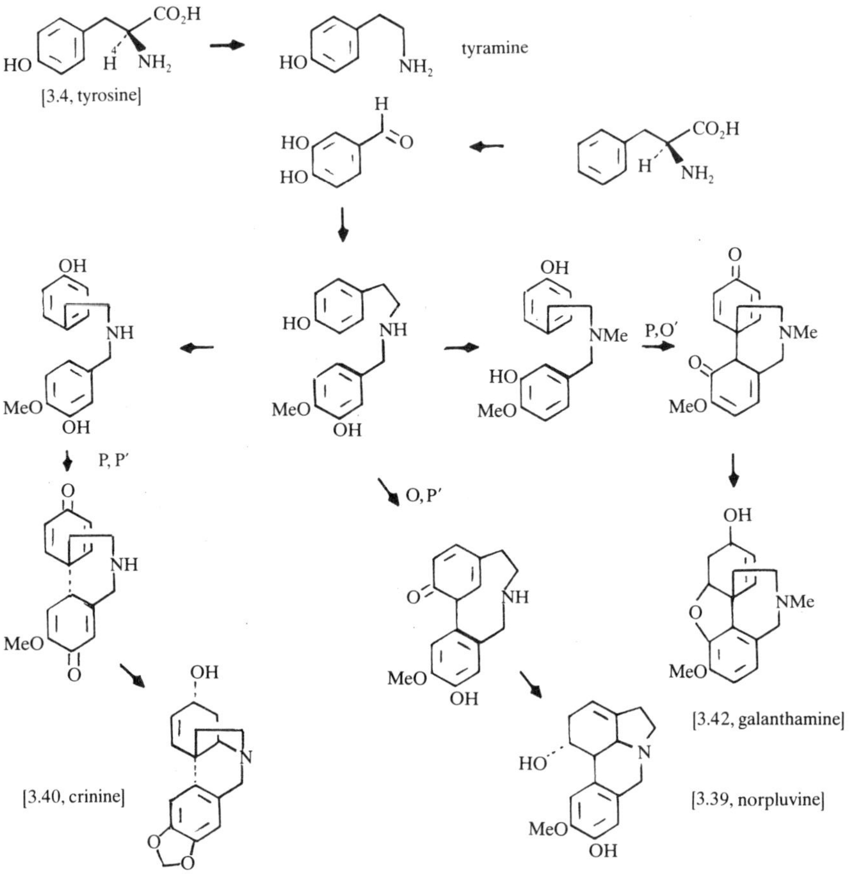

Scheme 3.7. Biosynthesis of isoquinoline alkaloids in the Amaryllidaceae.

oxidative cyclization of the N-methyl group of the precursor [3.28*b*], thus validating an early speculation of biogenetic theory.[1] The process is presumably analogous to the oxidative generation of the methylene dioxy function from a mono-O-methyl ether of catechol. Ultimately, both of these single carbon atoms are therefore derived from S-adenosyl methionine (SAM), which serves as a one-carbon donor in many biochemical reactions. These reactions are both shown in the sequence of steps leading from norlaudanosoline [3.27] through S-reticuline [3.28*b*] to the alkaloid berberine (Scheme 3.8).

As with the polyketides, many alkaloids are finally metabolized by sequences of reactions which lead to deep-seated modifications of the original precursor skeleton. These changes occur so as to effectively obscure the identity of the initial precursor. Typical of such metabolites are the benzophenanthridine alkaloids as, for example, chelidonine [3.45]. Some initial speculations favoured

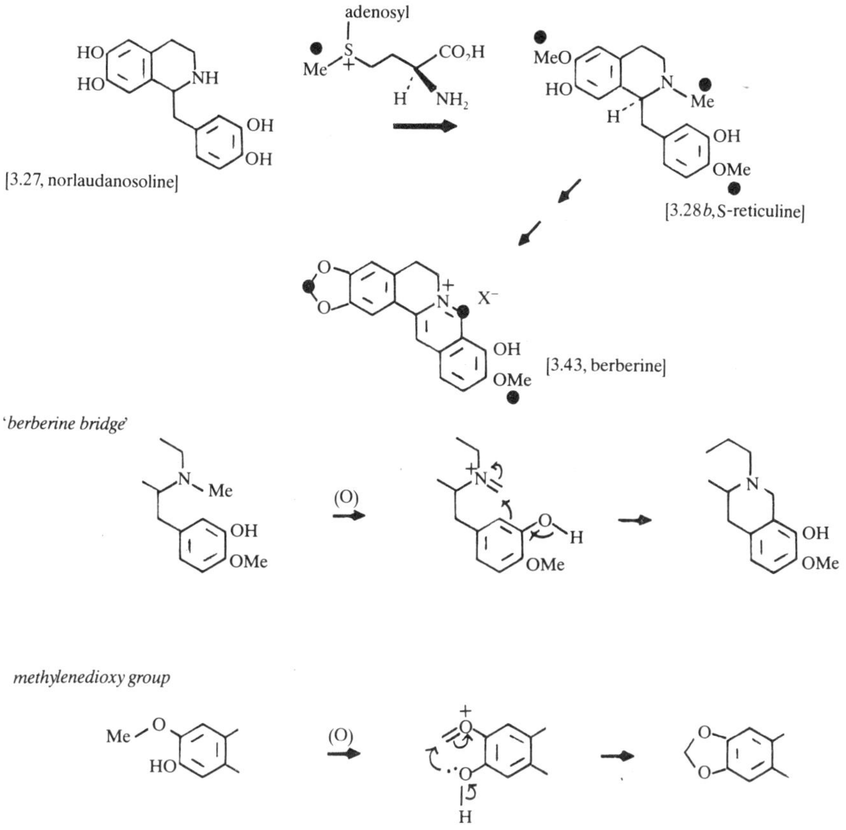

Scheme 3.8. Biosynthesis of berberine: biosynthetic origins of the 'berberine bridge' and the methylenedioxy group.[19]

the generation of this particular carbon–nitrogen skeleton in ways unrelated to other benzyl-tetrahydroisoquinoline alkaloids. Robinson argued otherwise, and subsequent brilliant experimentation[20] has supported this view. Tracer experiments have thus shown that chelidonine [3.45] is derived from (S)-reticuline [3.28b] via (S)-stylopine [3.44] in *Chelidonium majus*. The nature of these experiments has beautifully revealed the stereochemical detail of many of the processes in this pathway (Scheme 3.9). The phthalide isoquinoline alkaloids hydrastine [3.46] and protopine [3.47] are others derived by variations of this pathway.

Biogenetic theories have been remarkably successful in predicting the events which lead to the phenylethylamine derived alkaloids. Union of a phenylethylamine fragment such as tyramine or dopamine [3.25] with a further aromatic unit, gives rise to either the phenyl- or benzyl-tetrahydroisoquinoline group of alkaloids. Analogous condensation with an aliphatic species leads[12] alternatively

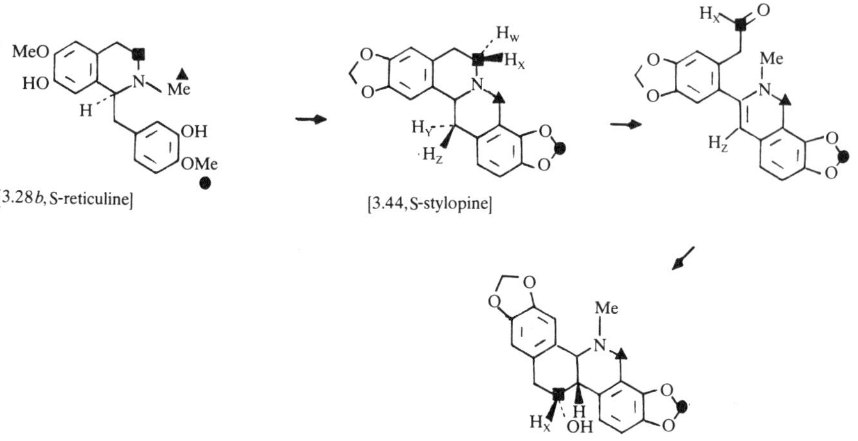

[3.28b, S-reticuline]

[3.44, S-stylopine]

[3.45, chelidonine]

Scheme 3.9. Biosynthesis of chelidonine in *Chelidonium majus*.[20]

to alkaloids such as pellotine ([3.38] pyruvate) and lophocerine ([3.49] meva-lonate). Laboratory stimulation, under physiological conditions of pH and temperature of this initial condensation, has given rise to a number of important biomimetic syntheses. Bearing in mind the inherent dangers in pressing laboratory analogies too far, they nevertheless illustrate the mechanistic viability of the bio-synthetic proposals.

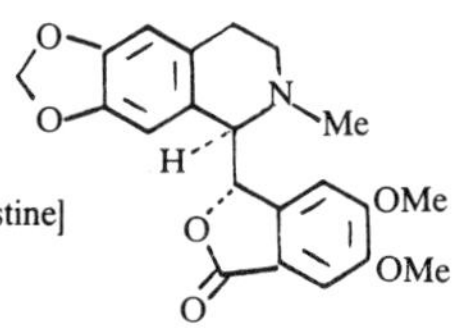

[3.46, hydrastine]

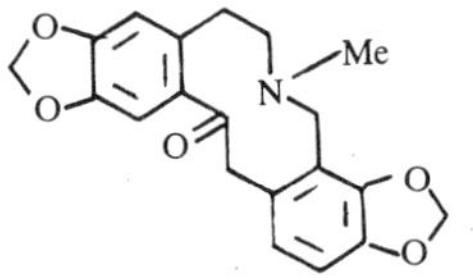

[3.47, protopine]

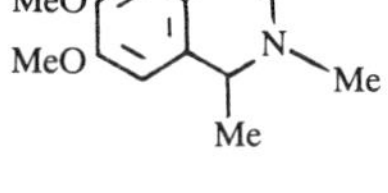

[3.48, pellotine]

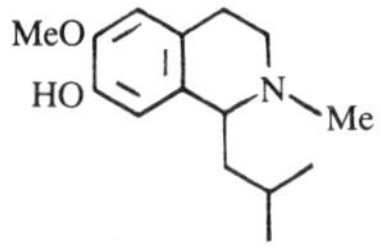

[3.49, lophocereine]

Typical of these biogenetically-modelled syntheses is that of the alkaloid salsolin (Scheme 3.10).

A great concentration of effort has also quite naturally been given over to attempts to mimic the many oxidative phenolic couplings which are implied[8] as playing crucial roles in the development of particular pathways of biosynthesis amongst the phenylethylamine derived alkaloids (*vide supra*). Thus oxidation of laudanosoline [3.50] with 0.2 M ferric chloride gives a 65 per cent yield of

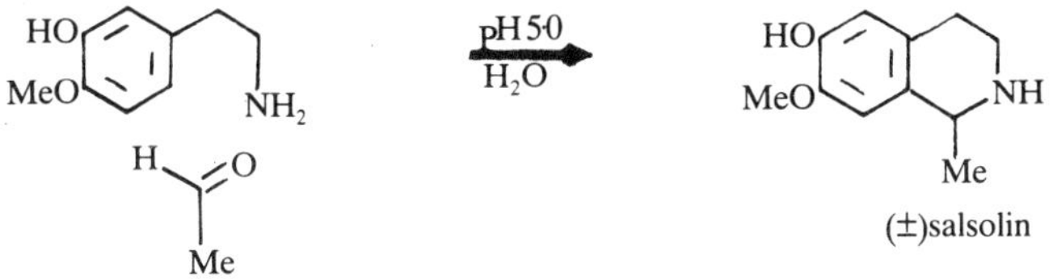

Scheme 3.10. Biomimetic synthesis of salsolin.[21]

the aporphine [3.51]. This particular reaction is critically dependent on the concentration of the ferric salt and with 0.02 M solutions the pyrrocoline [3.52] is formed. Battersby[22] also successfully incorporated an oxidative cyclisation of (±)-orientaline [3.36] with alkaline ferricyanide in a successful biomimetic synthesis of the *Papaver* alkaloid isothebaine [3.37] (Scheme 3.12).

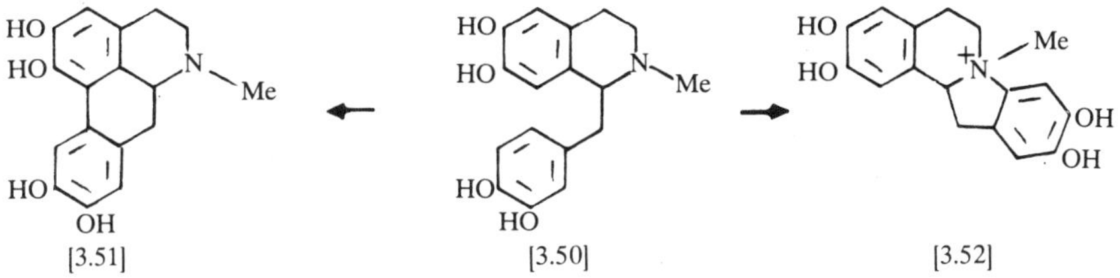

Scheme 3.11. Oxidation of laudanosoline.

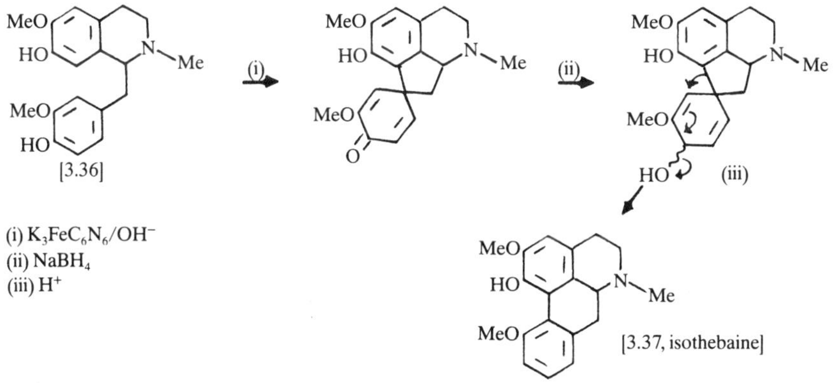

(i) $K_3FeC_6N_6/OH^-$
(ii) $NaBH_4$
(iii) H^+

Scheme 3.12. Biomimetic synthesis of (±)-isothebaine.[22]

3.5.2 *Indole alkaloids*

Finally, in this review of the commanding heights of alkaloid biosynthesis, brief reference is made to the origins of some of the indole alkaloids. One of the simplest modifications of the amino-acid tryptophan [3.5] is its conversion to gramine [3.53] the barley alkaloid—C-2 and the carboxyl group are lost but the amino-nitrogen is retained. Similarly, the structural resemblance of tryptophan to other alkaloids [3.54] [3.55] is readily apparent by inspection.

[3.5, tryptophan]

[3.53, gramine]

[3.54, psilocybin]

[3.55, harman]

By contrast, the biosynthetic story which lies behind the terpenoid indole alkaloids—the *Corynanthe-Strychnos, Aspidosperma* and *Iboga* types—is a complex and intricate one, with many of the features of the best 'whodunit'. Much of the biogenetic speculation has been ingenious, not to say original, and occasionally has given rise to controversy. Only one theory[23] has been found to stand the test of detailed experimental scrutiny.[24]

The number of known indole terpenoid alkaloids has increased sharply over the last twenty years. Some 600 examples were recorded in the mid-1960s, and over a thousand structures are now known in this the most widely-found group of plant alkaloids. A tryptamine residue (derived from tryptophan) appears invariant, and the bewildering structural variation is derived by the addition of a C_9-C_{10} unit attached to the tryptamine. It is the biosynthetic origins of this C_9-C_{10} fragment which has occasioned such prolific speculation and experimentation.[23,24]

Three major groupings of the indole terpenoid alkaloids may be discerned and these correspond to three principal arrangements of the C_9-C_{10} skeleton (Fig. 3.9). In those alkaloids where only nine skeletal carbon atoms are found attached to the tryptamine residue, it is invariably the carbon atom (─┼─) which is lost from the original C_{10} unit. The only biogenetic hypothesis in accordance with the subsequent experimental work is that due to Thomas and Wenkert.[23] This suggested a relationship of the C_9-C_{10} unit to the cyclopentane monoterpene skeleton. Figure 3.9 shows formally how the *Corynantheine–Strychnine* C_9-C_{10} unit [3.56] could be derived by cleavage of the cyclopentane ring. Likewise, the C_9-C_{10} units of the *Aspidosperma* [3.67] and *Iboga* [3.58] may be (in principle) elaborated by further appropriate bond fissions (⌒⌒) and new bond formations (⌒↴) from the intermediate [3.56] (Fig. 3.9). Proof of this attenuated relationship to the acyclic monoterpenes geraniol/nerol has been amply confirmed by various isotopic tracer experiments such as the incorporation of 3R-mevalonic acid and 2-^{14}C-geraniol (as its pyrophosphate) into the various terpenoid indole

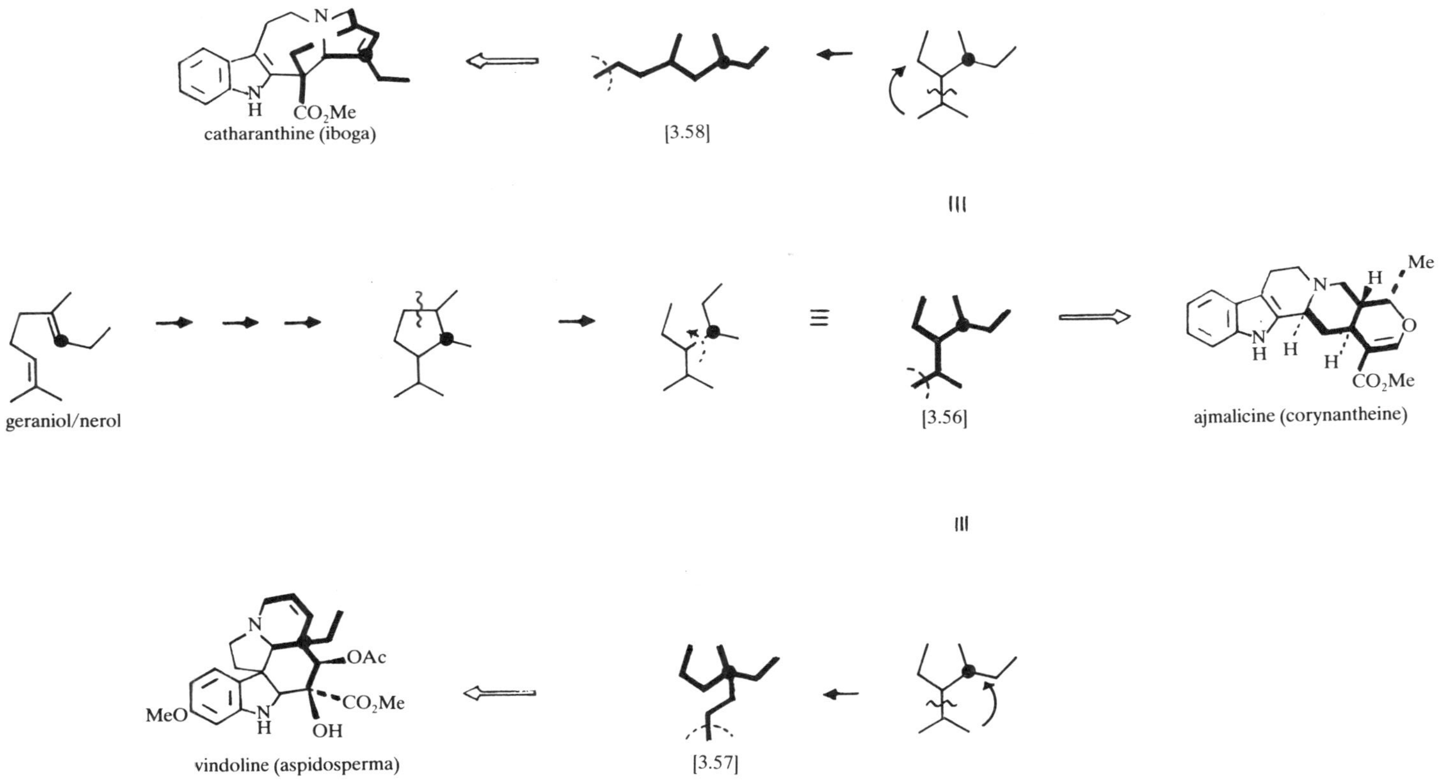

Fig. 3.9. Structural relationships in the indole terpenoid alkaloids: biosynthetic relationship to geraniol.[24]

alkaloids in *Vinca rosea* in the manner and pattern predicted by the hypotheses (Fig. 3.9).

Final identification of the C_9-C_{10} unit, which condenses with tryptamine [3.64] to furnish the terpenoid alkaloids, as the aldehyde secologanin [3.58] was made possible by the contemporaneous discovery of the structure of the Ipecachuana alkaloid [3.60]—ipecoside.[24] Biogenetic considerations suggested ipecoside [3.60] was formed by condensation of dopamine [3.25] with secologanin [3.58]. Moreover, extrapolating these same biogenetic arguments, the indole terpenoid alkaloids may be seen to be derived by an analogous condensation of tryptamine [3.60] with secologanin [3.58].

[3.58, secologanin]

[3.60, ipecoside]

Subsequent experimentation[25] established the biosynthetic sequence to secologanin [3.58] from geraniol/nerol via deoxyloganin [3.61] and loganin [3.62] in *Catharanthus roseus*. In addition, it was further demonstrated that both [3.61] and [3.62] are normal constituents of the same plant.

Contrary to the conclusions of tracer experiments, enzymic studies point[26] to strictosidine [3.63] as the first-formed intermediate which arises from the consensation of tryptamine [3.64] and secologanin [3.58]. The intermediate [3.63] is then converted *via* cathenamine to ajmalicine. *Corynanthe* alkaloids such as ajmalicine are the simplest structural variants of the strictosidine skeleton (Scheme 3.13). Numerous efforts have been made to clarify the steps to the various 'rearranged' alkaloids. The following sequence appears to be firmly established: Corynanthe → Corynanthe/Strychnos → Aspidosperma → Iboga alkaloids and the intermediate geissoschizine [3.65] is an important compound in these further conversions[27] of the strictosidine molecule [3.63].

3.6 Amino-acid metabolites—Penicillins and cephalosporins

Secondary metabolites containing the elements of two or more amino-acid structures are of frequent microbial occurrence; many possess antibiotic activity. Typical examples are shown in Fig. 3.10. Besides the amino-acids normally encountered in proteins, these metabolites may contain unusual non-protein amino-acids, those with irregular stereochemistry (e.g. D-configuration

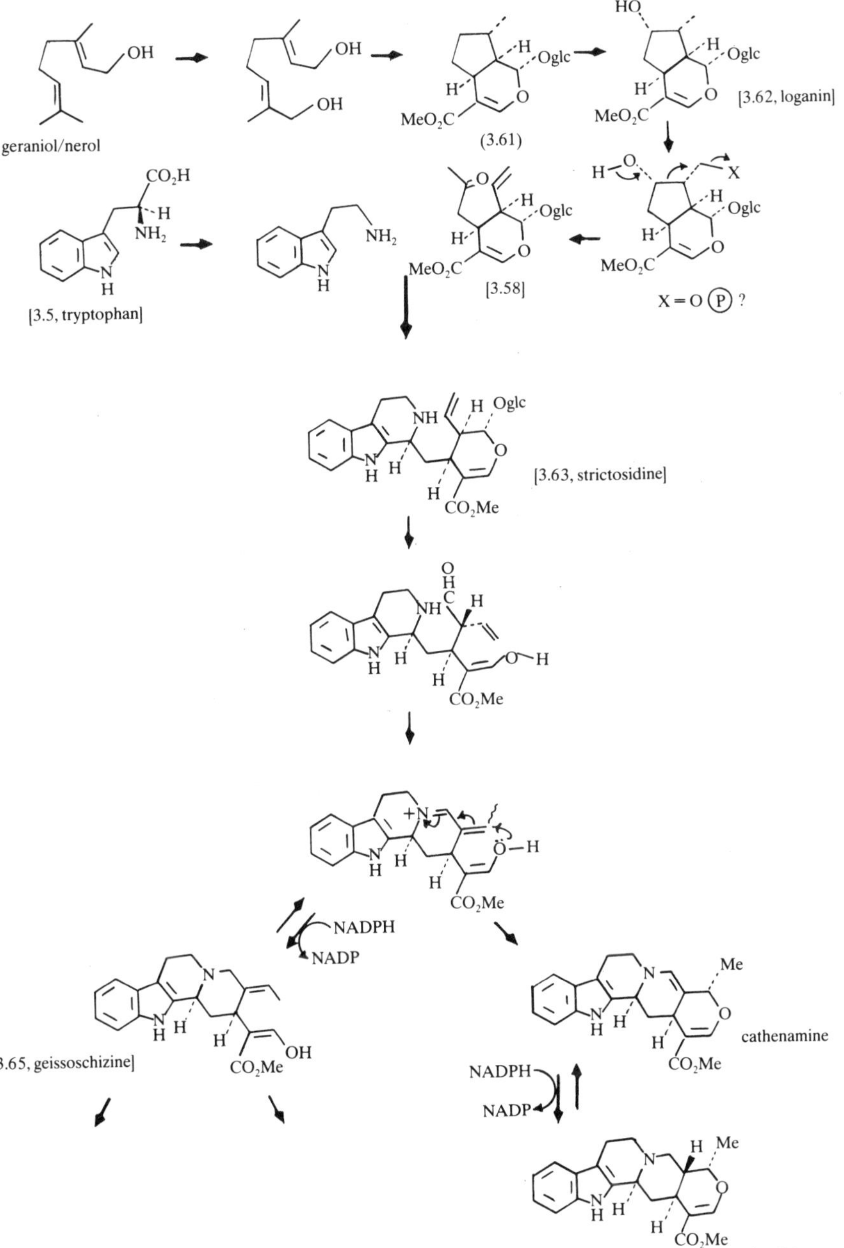

Scheme 3.13. Biosynthesis of ajmalicine.

at α-centre), and acids modified by methylation, hydroxylation, addition of the ubiquitous mevalonic acid derived terpenoid $(C_5)_n$ units, and other more extensive structural changes. Considerable attention has been devoted to the mechanism of generation of the D-α-amino configuration in the peptide antibiotics. A wholly satisfactory rationale for this process has not yet been formulated, but it is known that the α-keto acid is not an intermediate, and that the α-amino group is retained in the conversion from the L-amino-acid. Peptide secondary metabolites of the type shown in Fig. 3.10 are usually formed as mixtures of closely-related compounds, but with one product predominating. The presence of particular amino-acids in the nutrient medium often appears to strongly influence the nature of the product profile. However, so far as can be judged, the synthesis of peptides of this class is not analogous to that of proteins and is not ribosomally based.

Historically, because of their early discovery, scientifically, because of the interest and problems they continue to stimulate, and medically, because of their wide therapeutic application, the penicillins (and cephalosporins) are the pre-eminent examples of this class of secondary metabolite. They are, moreover, a classic illustration of the use man has made of the synthetic capabilities of micro-organisms.[28] Modern strains of *Penicillium chrysogenum* are capable of producing up to 100 000 units/ml of penicillin in a submerged culture, and by the mid-1970s the pharmaceutical industry was producing 7000 tons of penicillins annually. Although the discovery in 1929 by Fleming of the β-lactam antiobiotics is a tale which has become fixed in the popular mythology of science, it is now clear that for at least sixty years there had been a growing awareness of the antibacterial properties of *Penicillium* sp.

Penicillium chrysogenum produces a number of different penicillins. These differ in the nature of the non-polar side-chains, and this in turn is determined by the particular side-chain precursor which is added to the fermentation medium. Mono-substituted acetic acids are the most effective precursors. Over a hundred penicillins may be produced by such fermentations, but of these only benzyl-penicillin (penicillin G [3.66], $R = PhCH_2CO$-) and penicillin V([3.66] $R = PhOCH_2CO$-) have wide clinical utility. It has been suggested that penicillin production in these cases can be regarded as a detoxification of carboxylic acids such as phenylacetic acid by linkage to 6-amino-penicillanic acid [3.73]. Two other products may accumulate in the *Penicillium* type of fermentation, especially when the availability of the side chain precursor is limited—namely, isopenicillin N [3.72] and 6-amino-penicillanic acid (6-APA [3.73]).

The organism *Cephalosporium acremonium* shows a different pattern of metabolism. Penicillin N [3.74] is the sole penicillin derivative found, but, in addition, a number of cephalosporins [3.67] are produced. Mutants of *C. acremonium* have not been reported which metabolise cephalosporins *but not* penicillin N. In contrast, mutants blocked in cephalosporin production may or may not metabolize pencillin N [3.74]. In fermentations of the *Cephalosporium* type, increase in oxygen tension leads to a higher production of cephalosporins and a concommitant lower production of penicillin N. All of these observations are consistent with the hypothesis that the cephalosporins are produced *after* penicillin N in *Cephalosporium* fermentations.

In spite of the extensive efforts over the past two to three decades, some features of the detailed biosynthetic pathway to the β-lactam antibiotics—the

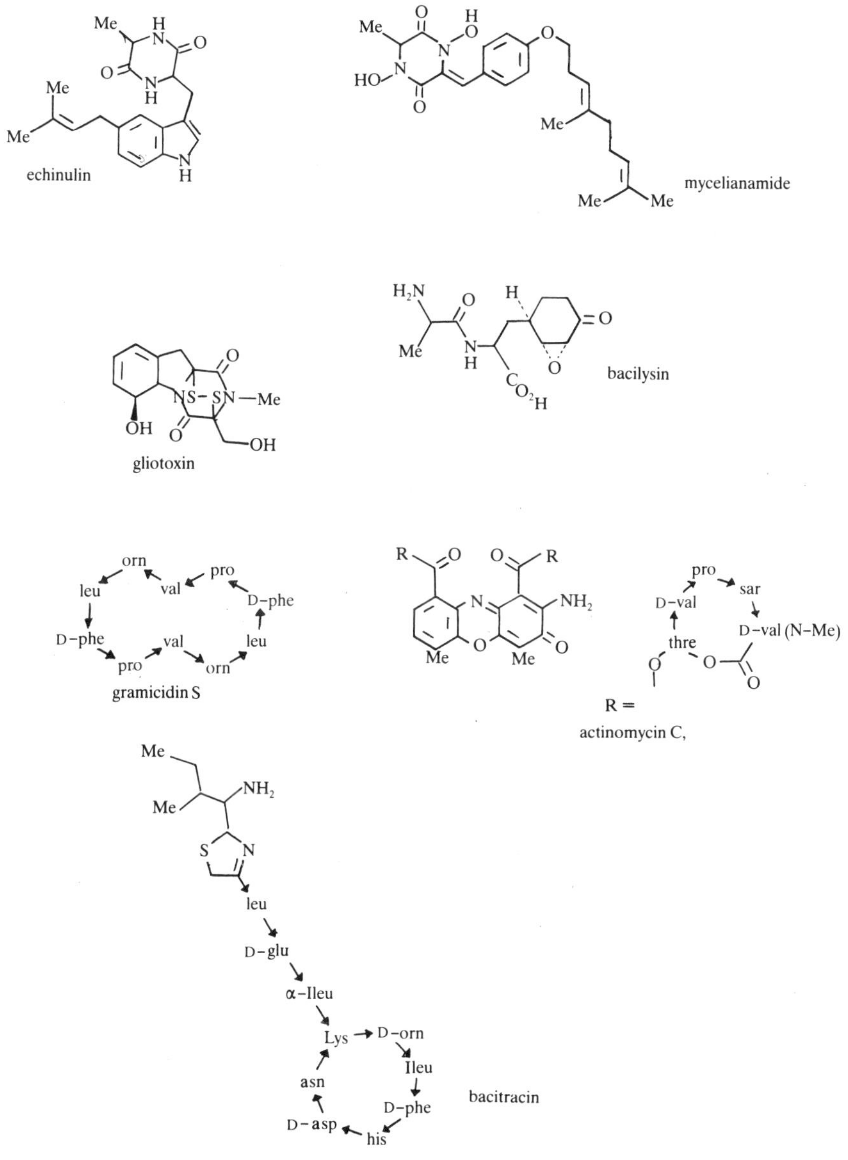

Fig. 3.10. Some modified peptide secondary metabolites.

archetypal antibiotics—are still uncertain.[29] The problem has been an outstanding one of biosynthesis. Its final and total solution has remained a tanta-
lizing but elusive prize. The evident structural relationship of the bicyclic penam
[3.66] and 3-cephem [3.67] nucleii to the amino-acids L-valine [3.68] and
L-cysteine [3.69] has been established by innumerable tracer experiments.[29]

[3.66, penam] [3.69, cysteine] [3.68, valine] [3.67, 3-cephem]

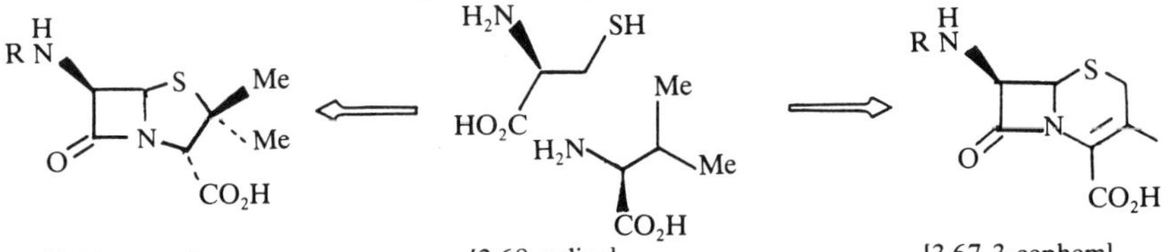

As each successive theory adumbrated to account for the formation of the fused
β-lactam structures [3.66] [3.67] was undermined and then found to be un-
tenable, these tracer experiments moved to increasing degrees of elegance and
sophistication in order to determine the fate of individual atoms in the metabolic conversions. Typical of these experiments are those[30] carried out to
illuminate the manner in which the diastereotopic methyl groups of L-valine
[3.68] are incorporated into the penam and 3-cephem nuclei. The tracer
employed was ^{13}C; syntheses of 3S and 3R (^{13}C-methyl) valine are depicted
(Fig. 3.11). Incorporation of the two isotopically-labelled samples of valine and
^{13}C n.m.r. analysis of the derived metabolites, showed that assimilation into the
penicillins proceeds with *retention* of configuration at C-3 of valine and into the
cephalosporins, with the 3S-methyl group ultimately appearing as a ring carbon
atom.

In 1960, Arnstein and his collaborators reported[31] the isolation from the
mycelium of *Penicillium chrysogenum* of a tripeptide δ-(α-aminoadipyl)-
cysteinylvaline (ACV) which was later characterized as the L,L,D isomer [3.71].
Its synthesis starts at the N-terminus, probably with the formation of L-α-
aminoadipyl-L-cysteine, which then combines with L (rather than D)-valine.
Thus, at some later stage, the configuration of the valine residue must become
inverted to form the final tripeptide (ACV-L,L,D [3.71]). Arnstein suggested
that the tripeptide (ACV) was a probable intermediate in penicillin biosynthesis,[31] and the evidence which is now available agrees with this proposition. The mechanism of cyclization, which proceeds with retention of
configuration in each of the ring closures, remains a subject of speculation and
debate although it has engendered considerable scientific interest. It is well-
established that the peptide (ACV-L,L,D, [3.71]) is efficiently transformed
into isopenicillin N [3.72] by cell-free extracts of *Cephalosporium acremonium*,[32] and this is believed to be first-formed penicillin. The direct observation of this conversion using ^{13}C n.m.r. as a probe has recently been made.[33]

The ^{13}C-labelled tripeptide [3.71a] was incubated with the extract and the two ^{13}C signals (δ 26.7 and 31.8 p.p.m.) showed a uniform decrease in intensity as the reaction progressed. At the same time, there was a concomitant increase in intensity of the signals (δ 65.6 and 67.7 p.p.m.) of the corresponding carbon atoms of the penam nucleus as it was formed. No other enzyme-free intermediate reached concentrations sufficient to permit detection by this technique.

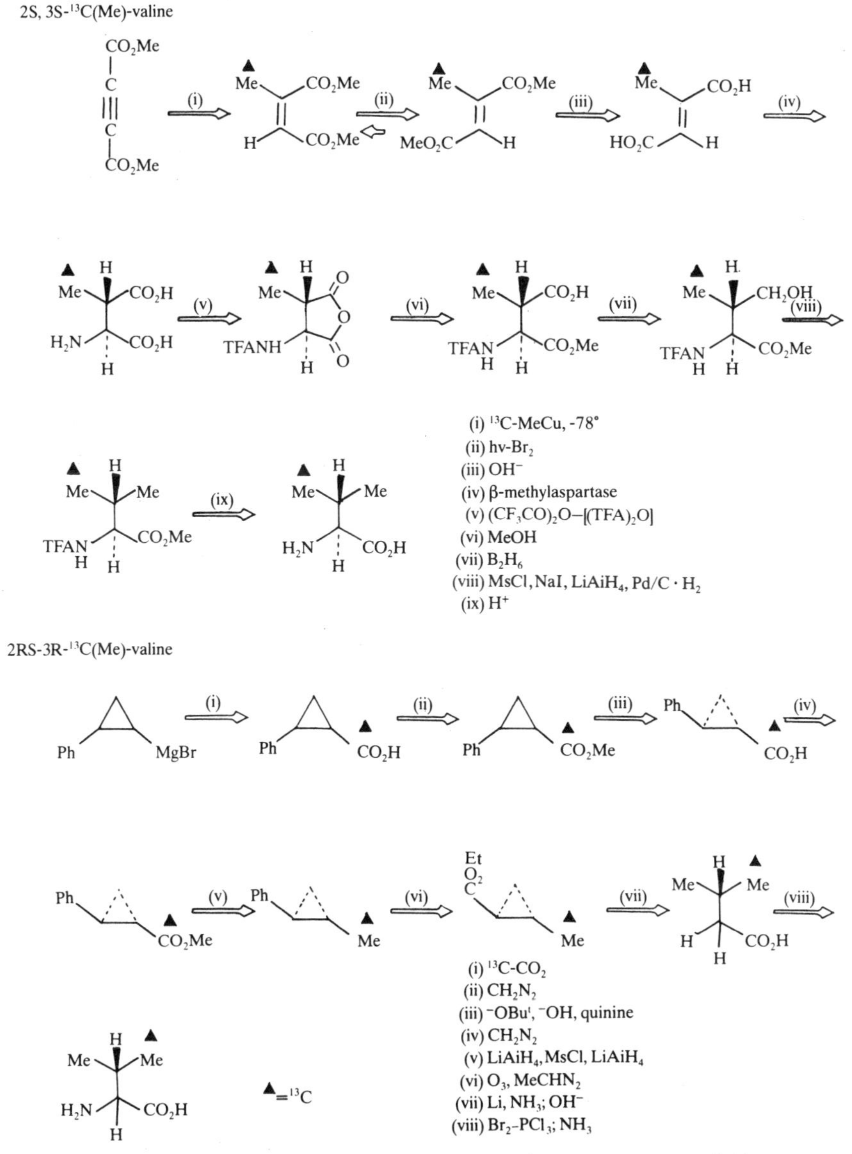

2S, 3S-^{13}C(Me)-valine

(i) ^{13}C-MeCu, -78°
(ii) hv-Br$_2$
(iii) OH$^-$
(iv) β-methylaspartase
(v) (CF$_3$CO)$_2$O−[(TFA)$_2$O]
(vi) MeOH
(vii) B$_2$H$_6$
(viii) MsCl, NaI, LiAiH$_4$, Pd/C · H$_2$
(ix) H$^+$

2RS-3R-^{13}C(Me)-valine

(i) ^{13}C-CO$_2$
(ii) CH$_2$N$_2$
(iii) $^-$OBu^t, $^-$OH, quinine
(iv) CH$_2$N$_2$
(v) LiAiH$_4$, MsCl, LiAiH$_4$
(vi) O$_3$, MeCHN$_2$
(vii) Li, NH$_3$; OH$^-$
(viii) Br$_2$-PCl$_3$; NH$_3$

$\blacktriangle = {}^{13}$C

Fig. 3.11. Synthesis of (3S)- and (3R)-^{13}C methyl-valines.[30]

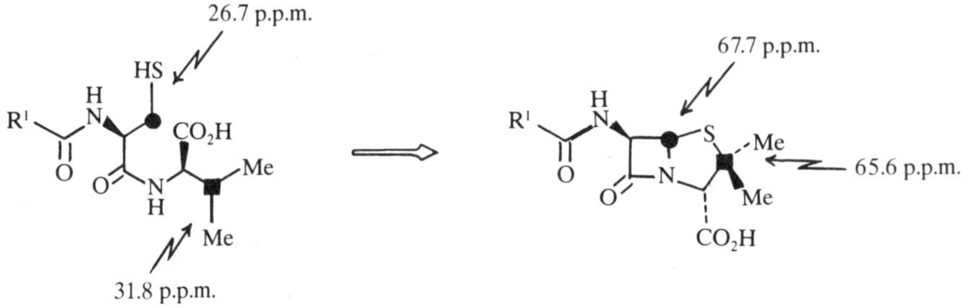

26.7 p.p.m.

67.7 p.p.m.

65.6 p.p.m.

31.8 p.p.m.

[3.71a]

[3.72, isopenicillin N]

The formation from (ACV [3.71]) of isopenicillin N [3.72] is believed to proceed via the initial formation of the β-lactam ring; particular attention has been devoted to the formation of the five-membered ring.

Baldwin and Wan have suggested a pathway which is in accord with the various chemical and stereochemical limitations imposed by biosynthetic experimentation. It is in addition supported by *in vitro* model experiments. They proposed that dehydrogenation of the enzyme-bound peptide [3.75] to the carbon radical [3.76]—possibly by an enzyme of the type able to hydroxylate saturated carbon—could result in an intramolecular trapping of the radical to yield the cyclized peptide (Scheme 3.14), as a diversion of the normal pathway of hydroxylation. Provided that ring closure is faster than rotation of the tertiary radical, then this mechanism satisfies all the known experimental facts.

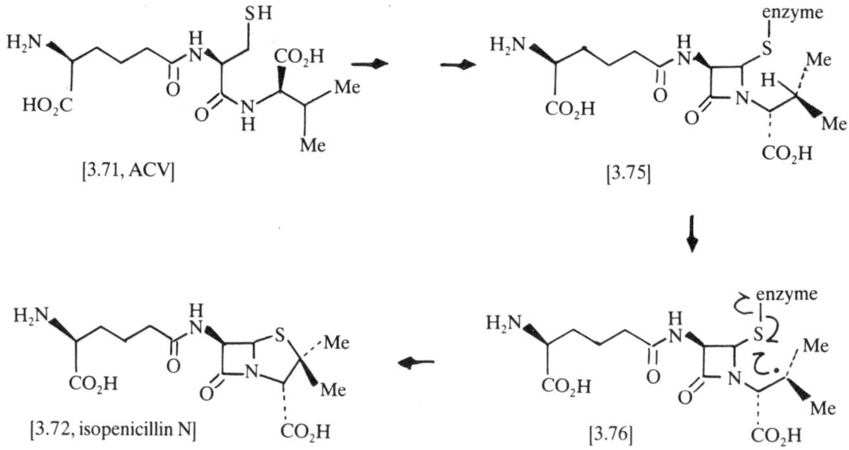

[3.71, ACV]

[3.75]

[3.72, isopenicillin N]

[3.76]

Scheme 3.14. Penicillin biosynthesis—carbon–sulphur bond formation.[34]

Enzymic conversion[35] (incubation with the purified isopenicillin-N synthetase, molecular weight 37 000, obtained from *Cephalosporium acremonium*) of the two modified tripeptide substrates [3.77] and [3.78], in which the D-valine residue of ACV is replaced respectively by [2R,3R]-3-^{2}H-α-amino butyrate and its diastereoisomer with the 3S configuration, gave, from both precursors, the same modified penicillin [3.80]. This observation suggests that isopenicillin-N synthetase is capable of forming the crucial C–S bond, either by retention [3.77] or by inversion [3.78], at the C-3 centre of the aminobutyrate residue. This result is in accord with the Baldwin postulate (Scheme 3.15), if it is assumed that rotation of the C-2–C-3 bond can occur in the active-site of the enzyme to generate a preferred conformation of the intermediate radical (Scheme 3.15) [3.79], which is then followed by an enzyme-directed radical coupling.

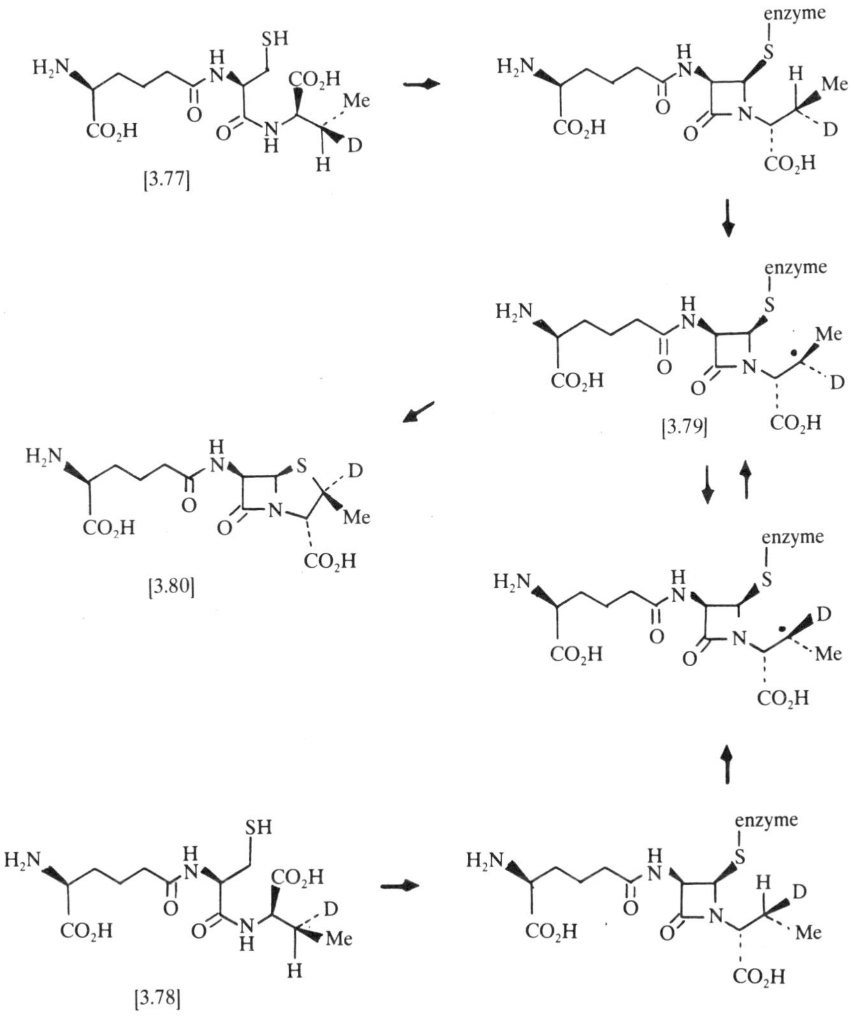

Scheme 3.15. Penicillin biosynthesis with modified substrates.[35]

Isopenicillin N [3.72] is therefore almost certainly the first penicillin synthesized from the tripepetide (ACV-L,L,D [3.71]). Since intact cells of *Cephalosporium acremonium* excrete penicillin N [3.74] with a D-α-aminoadipyl
side-chain, epimerization of the α-aminoadipyl group presumably occurs after
formation of the fused β-lactam ring system. Cell-free extracts of *Cephalosporium acremonium* mutants have now been obtained[34,36] which bring about
this same conversion, and also the transformation of isopenicillin N [3.72] to
deacetoxycephalosporin C [3.75].[36] Scheme 3.16 gives a summary of the pathways of penicillin and cephalosporin biosynthesis as they are presently understood.[29] A long-standing puzzle concerns the biosynthesis of the various
penicillins by fermentation, for example, penicillins G ([3.66] R = PhCH$_2$CO-)
and V ([3.67] R = PhOCH$_2$CO). In particular, at what stage is the new acyl
group introduced? Recent results strongly support the contention that isopenicillin N [3.72] is a normal precursor of penicillins with non-polar side-chains
produced by fermentation. Whether 6-amino-penicillanic acid [3.37] is a manda-
tory intermediate in this process still remains uncertain.

References

1. ROBINSON, R. *The structural relationships of natural products*, Clarendon
   Press, Oxford (1955).
2. WINTERSTEIN, E. and TRIER, G. *Die Alkaloide*. Borntraeger, Berlin
   (1910).
3. ROBINSON, R. *J. Chem. Soc.* **111**, 876 (1917).
4. ROBINSON, R. *J. Chem. Soc.* **111**, 762 (1917).
5. LEETE, E. *J. Am. Chem. Soc.* **84**, 55 (1962); *Tetrahedron Lett.* 1619
   (1964); *A. Rev. Pl. Physiol.* **18**, 179 (1967).
6. BATTERSBY, A. R., MARTIN, J. A., and BROCKMANN-HANSEN, E.
   J. Chem. Soc. (C) 1785 (1967).
   BATTERSBY, A. R., FOULKES, M. D., HIRST, M., PARRY, G. V., and
   STAUNTON, J. *ibid.* 210 (1968).
   BATTERSBY, A. R. *J. pure & appl. Chem.* **14**, 117 (1967).
7. BARTON, D. H. R., BHAKUNI, D. S., JAMES, R., and KIRBY, G. W. *J.
   Chem. Soc.* (C) 128 (1967).
8. BARTON, D. H. R. and COHEN, T. *Festschrift A. Stoll*, p. 117. Birkhaüser,
   Basle (1957).
   SCOTT, A. I. *Chem. Soc. Q. Rev.* 19, 1 (1965).
   TAYLOR, W. I. and BATTERSBY, A. R. *Oxidative coupling of phenols*.
   Marcel Dekker, New York (1967).
9. LARNER, J. *Intermediary metabolism and its regulation*. Prentice-Hall,
   New Jersey (1971).
10. SPENSER, I. D., in *Chemistry of the alkaloids* (ed. S. W. Pelletier), p. 669.
    Van Nostrand-Reinhold, London and New York (1970).
11. LEISTNER, E. and SPENSER, I. D. *J. Am. Chem. Soc.* **95**, 4715 (1973).

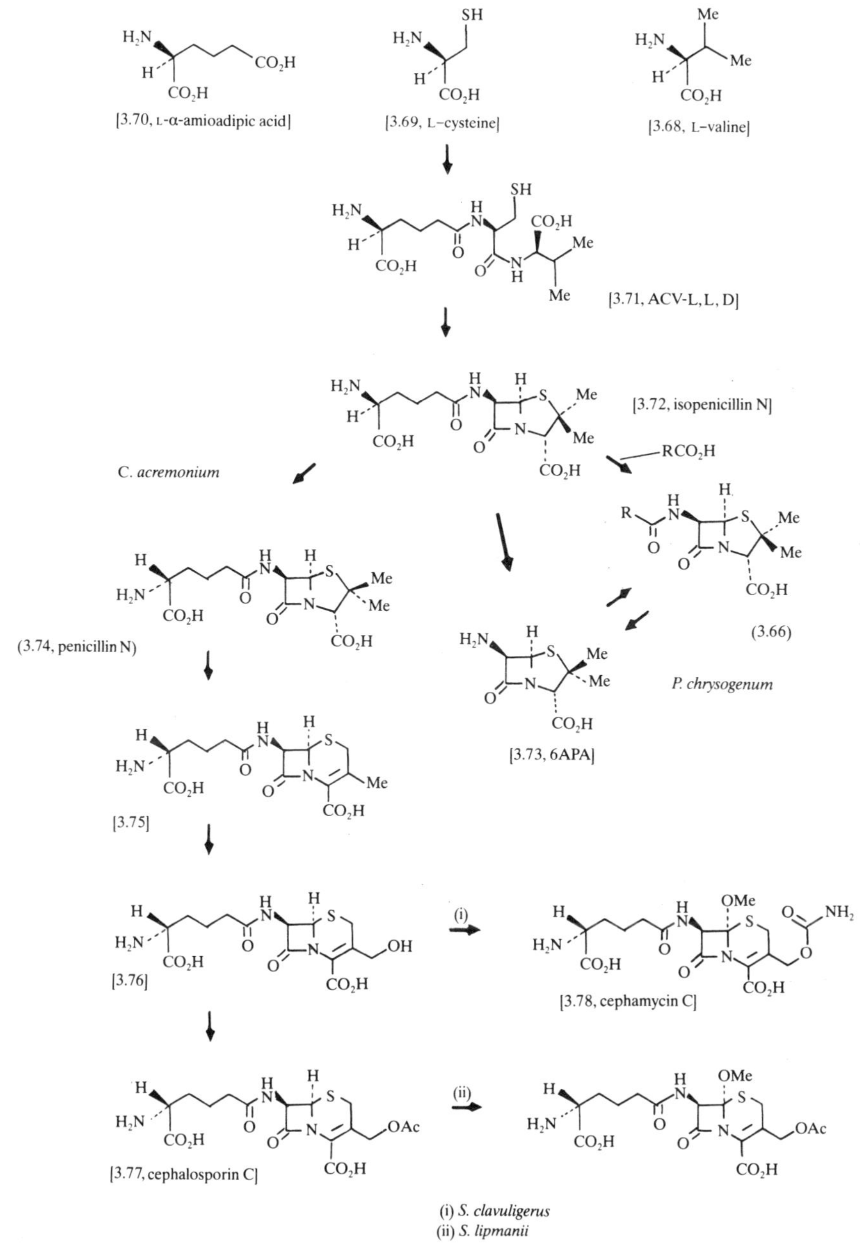

Scheme 3.16. Biosynthesis of penicillins and cephalosporins.[29]

SPENSER, I. D. and GOLEBIEWSKI, W. M. *J. Am. Chem. Soc.* **98**, 6726 (1976); *J. Chem. Soc., Chem. Commun.* 1509 (1983).

12. GEISSMAN, T. A. and GROUT, D. H. G. *Organic chemistry of secondary plant metabolism.* Freeman-Cooper, San Francisco (1969).

13. KHAN, H. A. and ROBINS, D. J. *J. Chem. Soc., Chem. Commun.* 554 (1981).
ROBINS, D. J. in *Progress in the chemistry of organic natural products* (ed. W. Herz, H. Grisebach and G. W. Kirby), Vol. 41, p. 115. Springer-Verlag, Vienna (1982).
ROBINS, D. J. *J. Chem. Soc., Chem. Commun.* 1289 (1982).

14. FRANCK, B. *Angew. Chem. int. edn* **18**, 429 (1979).

15. BARTON, D. H. R., BRACHO, R. D., POTTER, C. J., and WIDDOWSON, D. A. *J. Chem. Soc., Perkin Transactions 1*, 2278 (1974).
BATTERSBY, A. R., MACDONALD, E., MUNRO, M. H. G. and RAMAGE, R. *J. Chem. Soc., Chem. Commun.* 934 (1967).

16. BATTERSBY, A. R., MCHUGH, J. L., and RAMAGE, R. *J. Chem. J. Chem. Soc., Chem. Commun.* 985 (1971).

17. BATTERSBY, A. R., BROCKSTON, T. J., and RAMAGE, R. *J. Chem. Soc., Chem. Commun.* 464 (1969).

18. BATTERSBY, A. R., BINKS, R., BREUER, S. W., FALES, H. M., WILDMAN, W. C., and HIGHET, R. *J. Chem. Soc.* 1959 (1964).
BARTON, D. H. R., KIRBY, G. W., TAYLOR, J. B., and THOMAS, G. M. *J. Chem. Soc.* 4545 (1963).

19. BARTON, D. H. R., HESSE, R. H., and KIRBY, G. W. *Proc. Chem. Soc.* 267 (1963).
BATTERSBY, A. R., FRANCIS, R. J., HIRST, M., and STAUNTON, J. *Proc. Chem. Soc.* 268 (1963).
GEAR, J. R. and SPENSER, I. D. *Can. J. Chem.* 783 (1963).

20. BATTERSBY, A. R., FRANCIS, R. J., HIRST, M., RUVEDA, E. A., and STAUNTON, J. *J. Chem. Soc., Perkins Transactions 1* 1140 (1975); ibid. 1147 (1975).

21. KOVACS, O. and FODOR, G. *Chem. Ber.* **84**, 795 (1951).

22. BATTERSBY, A. R. and BROWN, T. H. *J. Chem. Soc., Chem. Commun.* 85 (1964).

23. THOMAS, R. *Tetrahedron Lett.* 544 (1961).
WENKERT, E. and BRINGI, N. V. *J. Am. Chem. Soc.* **81**, 1974 (1959).

24. BATTERSBY, A. R. *J. pure & appl. Chem.* **14**, 117 (1967).

25. BATTERSBY, A. R., HALL, E. S., and SOUTHGATE, R. *J. Chem. Soc.* (C) 721 (1969).
BATTERSBY, A. R., BYRNE, J. C., KAPIL, R. S., MARTIN, W. A., PAYNE, T. G., ARIGONI, D., and LOEW, P. *J. Chem. Soc.. Chem. Commun.* 951 (1968).
ESCHER, S., LOEW, P., and ARIGONI, D. *J. Chem. Soc., Chem. Commun.* 823 (1970).

BATTERSBY, A. R., BURNETT, A. R., and PARSONS, R. G. *J. Chem. Soc.* (*C*) 1187 (1969).

26. RUEFFER, M., NAGAKURA, N., and ZENK, M. H. *Tetrahedron Lett.* 1593 (1978).
   SCOTT, A. I., LEE, S.-L., and WAN, W. *Biochim. biophys. Res. Commun.* **75** 1004 (1975).
   STÖCKIGT, J., HUSSON, H. P., KAN-FAN, C., and ZENK, M. H. *J. Chem. Soc., Chem. Commun.* 164 (1977).
   STÖCKIGT, J. and ZENK, M. H. *J. Chem. Soc., Chem. Commun.* 642 (1977).
   STÖCKIGT, J., RUEFFER, M., ZENK, M. H., and HOYER, G.-A. *Planta Medica* **33**, 188 (1978).

27. BATTERSBY, A. R. and HALL, E. S. *J. Chem. Soc., Chem. Commun.* 793 (1969).
   STÖCKIGT, J. *J. Chem. Soc., Chem. Commun.* 1097 (1978).

28. SELWYN, S. *The beta-lactam antibiotics*, Hodder & Stoughton, London (1980).

29. O'SULLIVAN, J. and ABRAHAM, E. P. in *Antibiotics IV: Biosynthesis* (ed. J. W. Corcoran) Springer-Verlag, New York-Heidelberg-Berlin (1981).
   FAWCETT, P. A. and ABRAHAM, E. P. *Biosynthesis*, (ed. J. D. Bu'Lock), **4**, 248 (1976).

30. BALDWIN, J. E., NEUSS, N., NASH, C. H., LEMKE, P. A., and GRUTZNER, J. B. *J. Am. Chem. Soc.* **95** 3796, 6511 (1973).
   KLUENDER, H., SIH, C. J., BRADLEY, C. H., FAWCETT, P., and ABRAHAM, E. P. *J. Am. Chem. Soc.* **95**, 6149 (1973).

31. ARNSTEIN, H. R. V., ARTMAN, M., MORRIS, D., and TOMS, E. J. *Biochem J.* **76** 353 (1960).
   WOLFF, E. C. and ABRAHAM, E. P. *Biochem. J.* **76** 375 (1960).

32. O'SULLIVAN, J., BLEANEY, R. C., HUDDLESTON, J. A., and ABRAHAM, E. P. *Biochem. J.* **184**, 421 (1979).
   KONOMI, T., HERCHEU, S., BALDWIN, J. E., YOSHIDA, M., HUNT, N. A., and DEMAIN, A. L., *Biochem. J.* **184**, 427 (1979).

33. BALDWIN, J. E., JOHNSON, B. L., USHER, J. J., ABRAHAM, E. P., HUDDLESTON, J. A., and WHITE, R. L. *J. Chem. Soc., Chem. Comm.*, 1271 (1980).

34. BALDWIN, J. E. and WAN, T. S. *J. Chem. Soc., Chem. Commun.*, 249 (1979).

35. BALDWIN, J. E., ABRAHAM, E. P., ADLINGTON, R. M., MURPHY, J. A. GREEN, N. B., TING, H.-H., and USHER, J. J. *J. Chem. Soc., Chem. Comm.*, 1319 (1983).

36. SAYATILAKE, G. S., HUDDLESTON, J. A., and ABRAHAM, E. P. *Biochem. J.*, **194**, 645 (1981).
   BALDWIN, J. E., KEEPING, W., SINGH, P. D., and VALLEJO, C. A. *Biochem. J.*, **194**, 649 (1981).

4

PLANT PHENOLS

4.1 Introduction and L-Phenylalanine ammonia lyase (PAL)

The tissues of higher plants contain a unique but highly characteristic group of phenolic secondary metabolites.[1] Many—such as the hydroxycinnamic acids and their derivatives[2]—one suspects are found almost universally throughout the plant kingdom, whilst others have a more limited, but still wide, taxonomic distribution. Although, at first sight, there is a bewildering diversity of structures within the group, there is a common biogenetic theme which brings a coherence to their chemistry and biochemistry. In one way or another, most plant phenols are formed *via* the shikimate pathway of aromatic amino-acid metabolism— some from the intermediates along the pathway but the majority through the intermediacy of L-phenylalanine [4.1] and its conversion to *trans*-cinnamic acid (Scheme 4.1). This is a key reaction in phenolic biosynthesis in higher plants,[3] and it is reasonable to assume, from the available evidence, that the enzyme (PAL, *vide infra*), acts at a switching point in metabolism to divert L-phenylalanine from the general pool of amino-acids utilized for protein synthesis to the whole gamut of phenolic phenylpropanoids and associated metabolites (Scheme 4.1). In this sense, the phenolic substances of plants are clearly related to many plant alkaloids, since they possess a common biogenetic origin in one of the three aromatic amino-acids.

4.2 The phenylpropanoid pool and lignin biosynthesis

The enzyme—L-phenylalanine ammonia lyase[4] (PAL)—which catalyses the conversion of L-phenylalanine to *trans*-cinnamic acid (Scheme 4.1) has been characterized from numerous plants and some fungi, and its distribution has been extensively catalogued. Circumstantial evidence suggests that its presence and that of the corresponding L-tyrosine ammonia lyase[5] in the Gramineae (Scheme 4.1), may broadly be correlated with the ability of plants to synthesize phenylpropanoid compounds related to the polymeric lignins. The first-formed product following the action of PAL is *trans*-cinnamic acid (Scheme 4.1) and there is good reason to believe[6] that the various hydroxycinnamic acids— *p*-coumaric [4.2], caffeic [4.3], ferulic [4.4], and sinapic [4.5] acids are derived sequentially by successive hydroxylations and O-methylations (Scheme 4.1). The acids [4.2] [4.4] [4.5], once formed, are activated as their coenzyme A

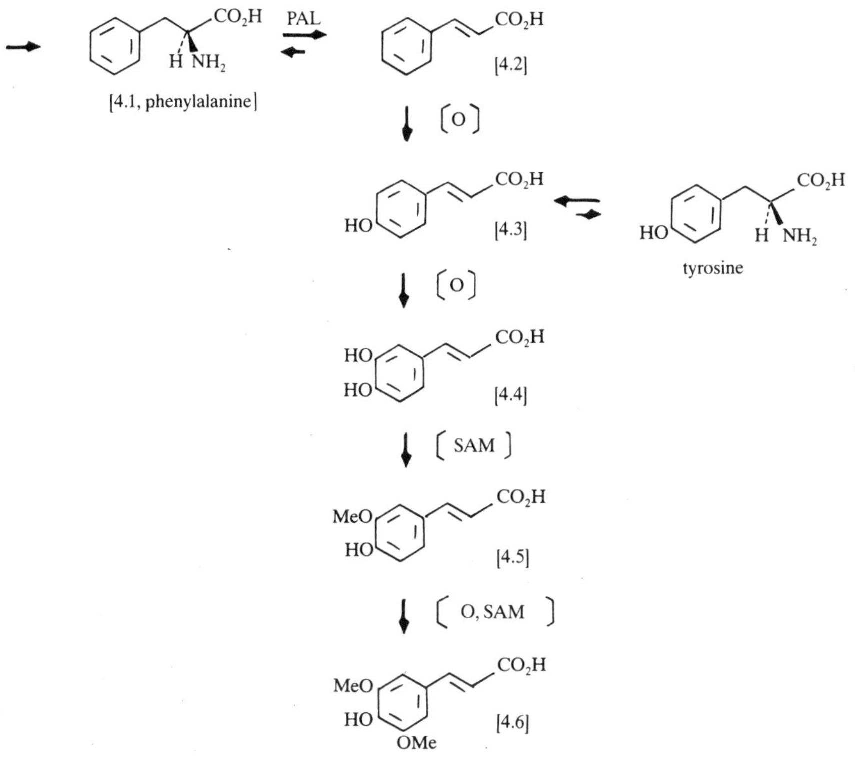

[4.1, phenylalanine] → [4.2] (PAL)

tyrosine → [4.3]

[4.3] → [4.4] ([O])

[4.4] → [4.5] (SAM)

[4.5] → [4.6] (O, SAM)

Scheme 4.1. Biosynthesis of the hydroxycinnamic acids.[6]

esters and reduced to the corresponding primary alcohols[7] which play direct roles in the synthesis of lignin *via*, it is presumed, a process of oxidative metabolism (Scheme 4.2). The formation and deposition of lignins in the plant cell wall is synonymous with the development of a vascular character. Although

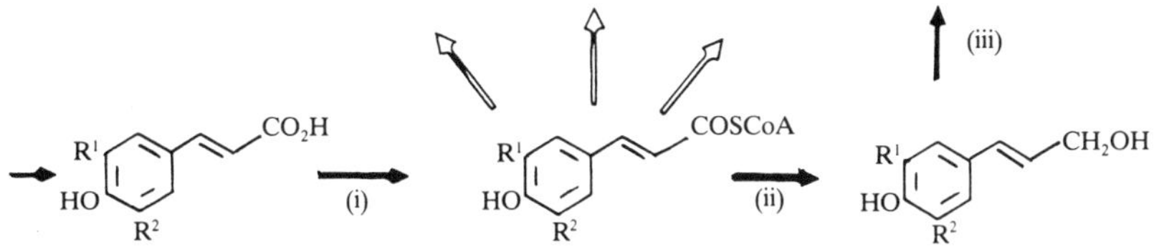

Lignins (iii)

$R^1 = R^2 = H$; p-coumaric
$R^1 = OMe, R^2 = H$; ferulic
$R^1 = R^2 = OMe$; sinapic

$R^1 = R^2 = H$; p-coumaryl
$R^1 = OMe, R^2 = H$; coniferyl
$R^1 = R^2 = OMe$; sinpayl

(i) ATP/CoASH;   (ii) NADPH;   (iii) [O]

Scheme 4.2. Biosynthesis of lignins.[7, 8]

the polymers themselves are inert, they nevertheless clearly serve a structural function, and the metabolic process which leads to their formation may therefore be regarded as a primary activity of the plant. The whole thrust of the diversion of L-phenylalanine [4.1] from the amino-acid pool may accordingly be viewed as biosynthetic activity directed towards the production of structural polymers of the lignin type.

4.3 Plant phenol biosynthesis

In a classic essay on the chemotaxonomy of plants, Bate-Smith[9] noted that in the leaves of vascular plants three classes of phenolic metabolite overwhelmingly predominate:

(i) esters, amides and glycosides of the hydroxycinnamic acids (principally those of p-coumaric, caffeic, ferulic and sinapic acids);

(ii) glycosylated flavonoids—principally those of kaempferol [4.7a], quercetin [4.7b], and myricetin [4.7c]; and

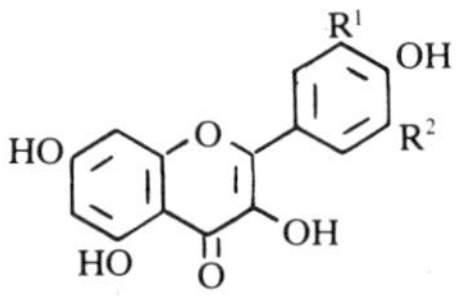

[4.7a, $R^1 = R^2 = H$, kaempferol]
[4.7b, $R^1 = H, R^2 = OH$, quercetin]
[4.7c, $R^1 = R^2 = OH$, myricetin]

(iii) proanthocyanidins—procyanidins [4.8a] and/or prodelphinidins [4.8b].

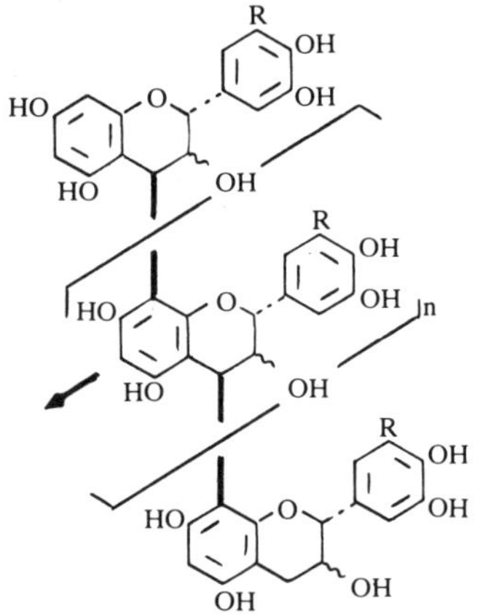

[4.8a, R = H; procyanidins]
[4.8b, R = OH; prodelphinidins]

The biosynthetic origin of these three classes of phenolic metabolite is generally assumed, although not explicitly stated, to be associated with the development of the ability to synthesize structural polymers of the lignin class. Very probably, the intermediate coenzyme A esters of the hydroxycinnamic acids in the enzymic reduction sequence (Scheme 4.2) form the points of biosynthetic departure to the various classes of phenolic metabolite [(i), (ii), (iii)—*vide supra*]. Viewed in this context, the role of some of these phenolic compounds may be simply as storage or shunt metabolites of the hydroxycinnamoyl coenzyme A esters—thus supporting the original suggestion of Bate-Smith[9] that the phenolic constituents in higher plants occupy a metabolic *cul de sac*.

Interception of the coenzyme A esters (Scheme 4.3) by sugars, polyols, or amines gives glycosides, esters, or amides of the various hydroxycinnamic acids.[2,7] These metabolites are ubiquitous in plant tissues, and it has often been suggested that this chemical association is a detoxification mechanism analogous, in many ways, to conjugation with glucuronic acid in mammals. It may also bring about enhanced solubility of the metabolite and lead to decreased sensitivity towards enzymic oxidation. Besides the hydroxycinnamic acids themselves and their derivatives, there is a wide variety of metabolites which are regarded as derived therefrom (Scheme 4.3). These have a much more restricted and more specialized distribution in the plant kingdom.[10,11]

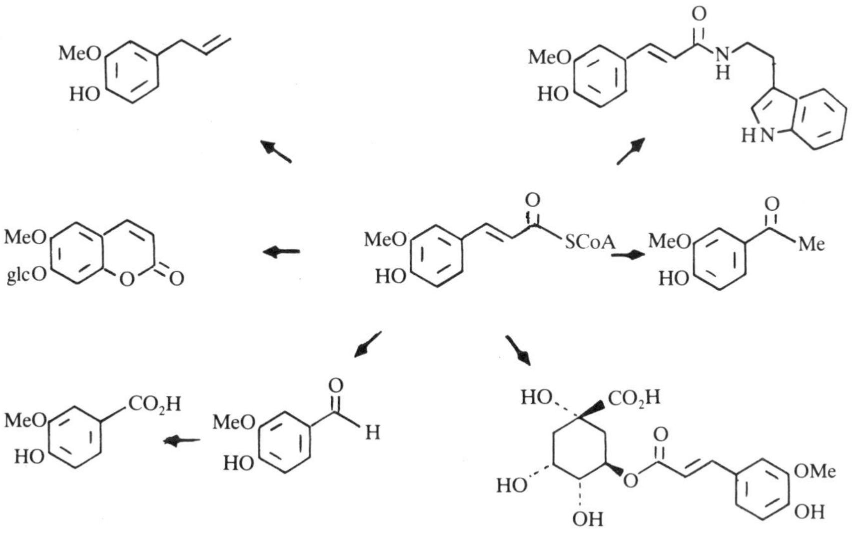

Scheme 4.3. Some metabolic transformations of the hydroxycinnamic acids[2,7] (e.g. ferulic acid).

The other key biosynthetic precursors in higher plant phenol biosynthesis are acetate/malonate units.[1,11] Several simple phenols and a number of plant quinones (Fig. 4.1) are derived directly from acetyl and malonyl coenzyme A *via* polyketide intermediates.[12] In this context, it is worth noting that this form of quinone synthesis represents just one of the possible pathways which operate in higher plants. One of the distinctive features of quinone biosynthesis in higher plants is the variety of different precursors which lead to quinones.[13] Other pathways derive from L-phenylalanine and shikimic acid with *o*-succinoyl benzoic acid. This latter pathway is responsible for the formation of a large number of both naphthoquinones (e.g. [4.9]) and anthraquinones (e.g. [4.10]).

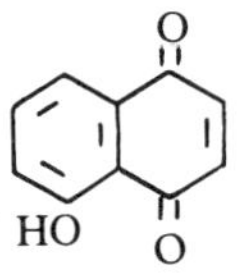
HO
O
O

[4.9, juglone]

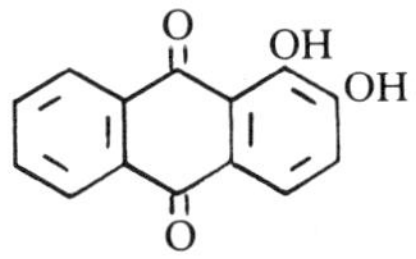
O
OH
OH
O

[4.10, alizarin]

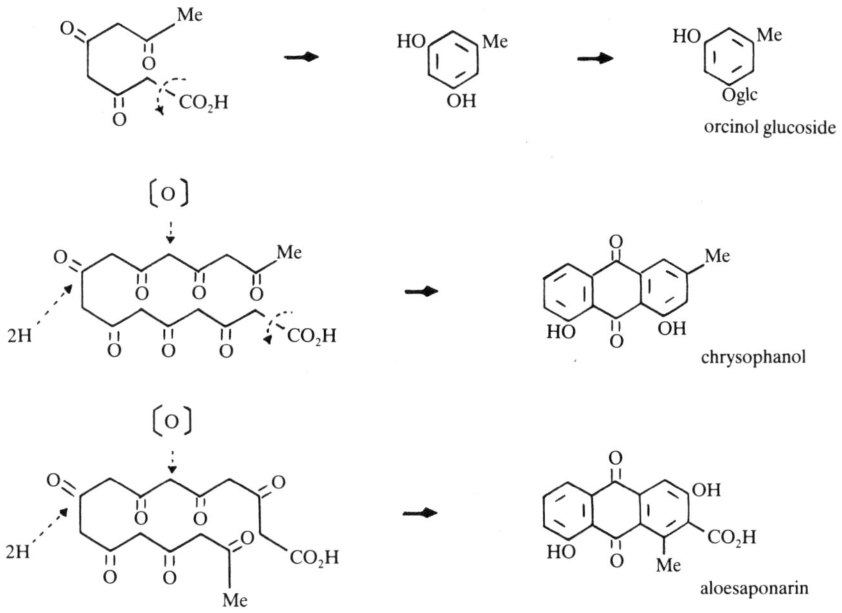
orcinol glucoside
chrysophanol
aloesaponarin
[O]
2H
CO2H
Me
HO
OH
Oglc

Fig. 4.1. Some polyketide metabolites in higher plants.[12, 13]

However, the major role of malonyl coenzyme A as a precursor in higher plant phenol metabolism is in its association with the hydroxycinnamoyl coenzyme A ($C_6.C_3$) unit or, less frequently, with the derived hydroxybenzoyl coenzyme A ($C_6.C_1$) unit to yield a range of distinctive secondary metabolites —flavonoids, stilbenes, xanthones, etc. (Scheme 4.4), which are unique to the plant kingdom.[14] Some of these possibilities were recognized theoretically by Birch and Donovan[15] in 1953 in their enunciation of the 'acetate hypothesis'.

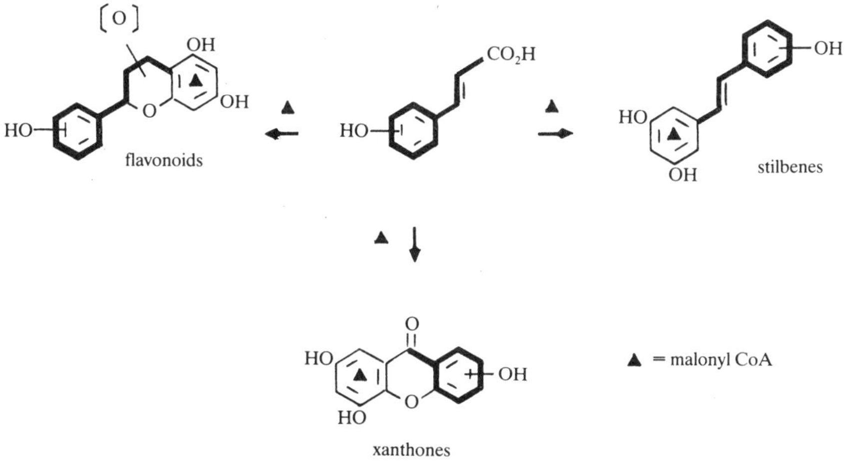

Scheme 4.4. Combined phenylpropanoid and acetate metabolism in higher plants.[14]

One speculation which they made was that alternative modes of cyclization of a common precursor such as [4.11], formed by the condensation of a hydroxycinnamic acid with three acetate units (malonyl coenzyme A), could give rise to the stilbene [4.14] on the one hand and the flavanone [4.13], via the chalcone [4.12], on the other (Scheme 4.5). This proposal accords with Robinson's earlier proposals,[16] and with chemical work in this area where it was noted that there were certain regularities in the patterns of hydroxyl and methoxyl substitution in the aromatic nuclei of plant phenols. Thus, in the flavonoid group of natural products, the oxygen-containing substituents (−OH, −OMe, Oglc) are, with few notable exceptions, in the meta positions in ring A (polyketide origin), but in the ortho relationship in ring B (hydroxycinnamic acid origin). Yangonin [4.15], an α-pyrone from *Piper methysticum*, was similarly envisaged as derived by the condensation of the phenylpropanoid precursor with two acetate units with subsequent cyclization on to oxygen rather than carbon (Scheme 4.5).

The total number of secondary phenolic metabolites obtained from plants is numerically impressive, but this is due less to a high degree of structural diversity than to the manner in which the parent carbon skeleton is 'chemically embroidered' (hydroxylated, alkoxylated, glycosylated, isoprenylated, etc.— Robinson's extra-skeletal processes).[16] The flavonoids, for example, comprise the largest single family of oxygen ring compounds occurring in Nature. They are responsible simply as plant pigments for the majority of the red, violet, and blue, and for several of the yellow and orange colours of flowers and other

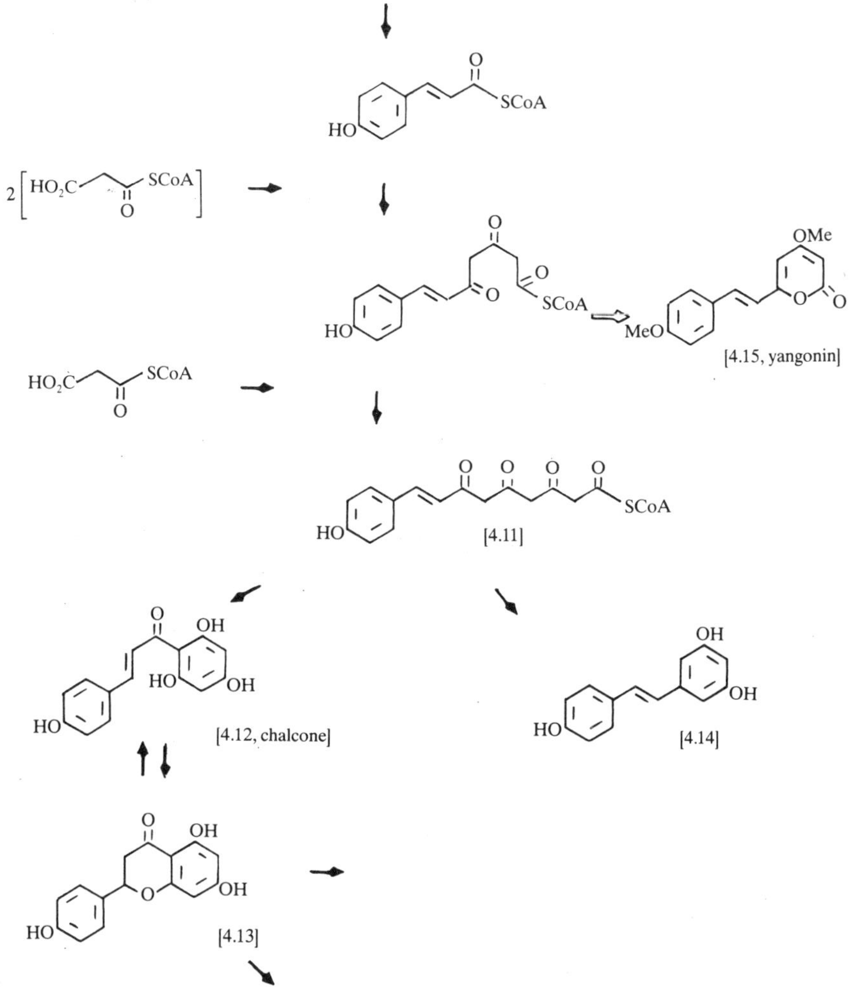

[4.15, yangonin]

[4.11]

[4.12, chalcone]

[4.14]

[4.13]

Scheme 4.5. Phenylpropanoid and acetate metabolism: biosynthetic proposals.[15]

plant tissues. The 2000 or so structures of the flavonoid class[1] are based on a diarylpropane carbon skeleton (C_{15}), and are conveniently divisible into (broadly) twelve groups according to the oxidation level of the oxygen heterocyclic ring and the position of phenyl substitution on the chroman ring. Two of the major classes of phenolic metabolite which predominate in the leaves of vascular plants,[9] noted above, flavonols [4.7] and the flavan-3-ol oligomers (proanthocyanidins [4.8]) represent two of these groups. Other commonly-occurring categories are the anthocyanidins, e.g. [4.16], and the flavonols, e.g. [4.17]. Isoflavonoids, e.g. [4.18] and [4.19], have a more limited taxonomic distribution in higher plants and are found primarily in the Leguminosae.

They all have in common the 3-phenyl chroman skeleton, whilst the neoflavonoids possess the 4-phenylchroman skeleton or a derivative thereof, e.g. [4.20]. The structures of many of the naturally-occurring flavonoids (Fig. 4.2) contain the characteristic C_5 isoprene units which are derived from γ,γ-dimethylallyl pyrophosphate or isopentenyl pyrophosphate. An additional structural variation of some interest is the flavonolignan class, in which a flavonoid has been biosynthetically intercepted by an additional phenylpropanoid unit, e.g. [4.21].

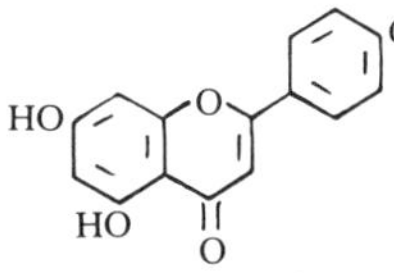

[4.17, apigenin]

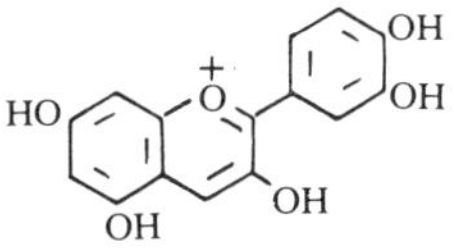

[4.16, cyanidin]

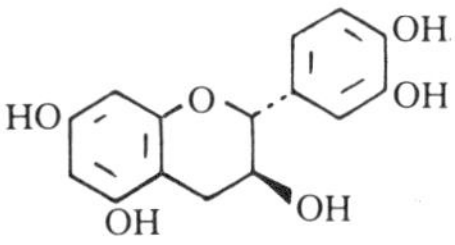

catechin

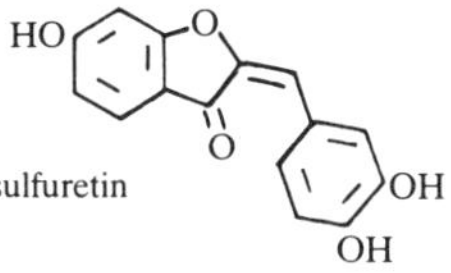

sulfuretin

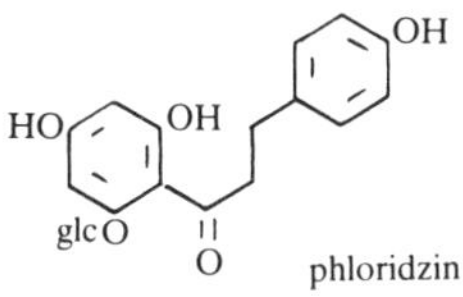

phloridzin

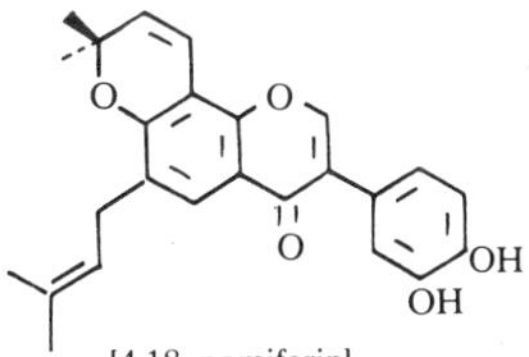

[4.18, pomiferin]

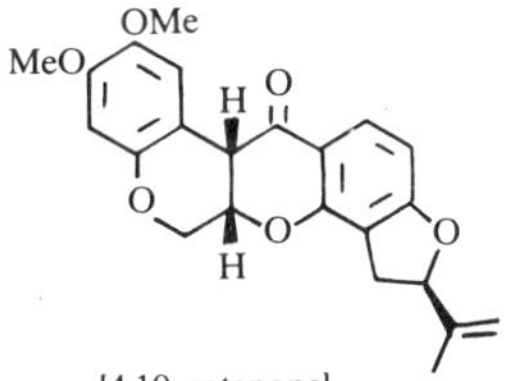

[4.19, rotenone]

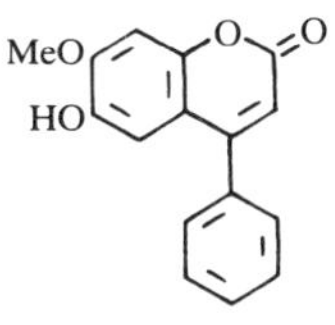

[4.20,dalbergin]

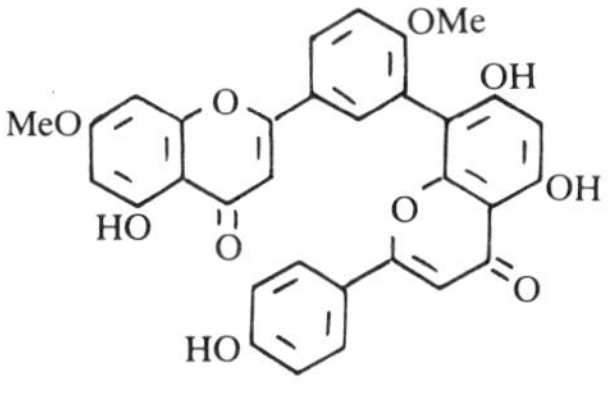

ginkgetin

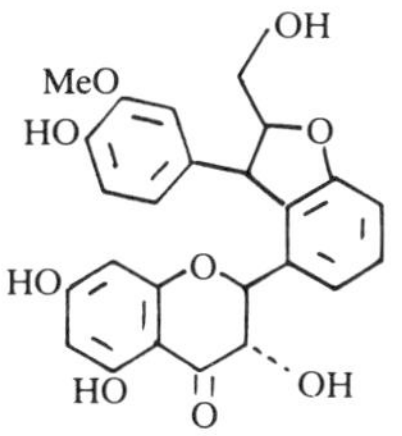

[4.21, silychristin]

Fig. 4.2. 'Flavanoid' metabolites.

Conventional isotopic tracer experiments have confirmed the correctness of Birch and Donovan's original hypothesis concerning the biosynthetic origins of the flavonoid (2-phenylchroman) and stilbene structures (Schemes 4.5. 4.6).[11,14] In many cases, however, the problems related to the formation of the individual types of flavonoid and the manner in which the oxidation level of the oxygen heterocyclic ring is established, are only partially solved. The postulated biosynthetic pathways are often based solely on good chemical analogy, but in these Grisebach and his collaborators have accorded dihydro-flavonols ([4.24] flavanonols) a key role[14,17] (Scheme 4.6). An important chemogenetic point which has been examined in detail in many studies of

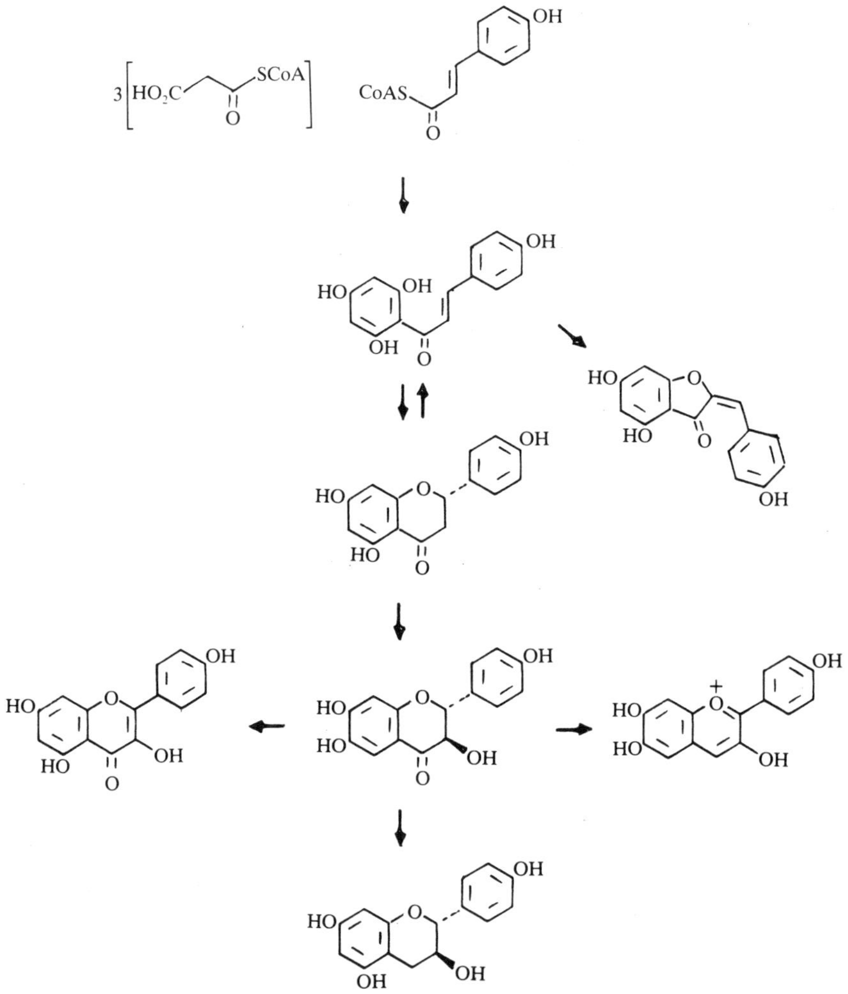

Scheme 4.6. Biosynthetic pathways to the flavanoids.[14, 17]

flavonoid biogenesis, is the stage at which the substitution pattern in ring B of the final product is established. The 'Zimtsaurestart' hypothesis of Hess[18] postulated that this occurred at the commencement of flavonoid biosynthesis by selection of the appropriate hydroxycinnamoyl coenzyme A ester from the phenylpropanoid pool (Scheme 4.1). On the other hand, the later substitution of the B ring (hydroxylation, methoxylation) at the stage of the C_{15} intermediate has been proposed by a number of workers on the basis of tracer experiments. The balance of evidence favours this possibility that synthesis of the intermediate chalcone [4.23] occurs initially *via* condensation of three molecules of malonyl coenzyme A with *p*-hydroxycinnamoyl coenzyme A [4.22], and that then further modification of ring B occurs at this stage[14] (Scheme 4.6).

The capacity to rearrange a flavonoid to an isoflavonoid structure is essentially limited to one phylogenetically-related group of plants, and is a molecular rearrangement which has attracted some attention and interest. It has generally been assumed, although as yet far from unequivocally proven, that the rearrangement occurs oxidatively via a 4-hydroxychalcone intermediate [4.25a,b]. Pelter's imaginative speculation[19] leads to the formation of a spirodienone [4.26] as the first-formed product of oxidation. Decomposition of this intermediate, either by protonation or by methylation (S-adenosyl-methionine, SAM) would yield four isoflavones [4.27a,b] [4.28a,b]. These are then envisaged as precursors of most, if not all, of the naturally-occurring isoflavonoids[20] (Scheme 4.7). Isotopic tracer experiments support the overall features of the molecular rearrangement.[20]

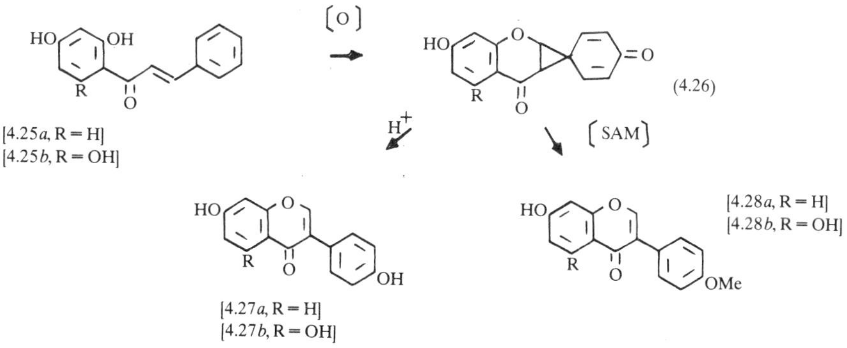

Scheme 4.7. Biosynthesis of isoflavones: 1,2-aryl migration.[19, 20]

Several phytoalexins (*vide infra*) possess isoflavonoid structures, and their synthesis in certain plants may be induced by appropriate chemical treatment or fungal infection. This has aided biosynthetic experimentation in this field, since the postulated precursor may then be administered to the plant at the stage of maximal synthesis. High incorporations (e.g. 1–10 per cent) into iso-flavonoid structures of isotopically-labelled precursors may then be possible.

This has recently permitted the use of ^{13}C as an isotopic tracer to study iso-flavonoid biosynthesis. Normally this has been difficult, if not impossible, to achieve because of the generally low levels of precursor incorporation which may be achieved with plants. Sodium 1,2-$^{13}C_2$ acetate [4.29] was fed to $CuCl_2$ treated pea plants (*Pisum sativum*) and the phytoalexin pisatin [4.30] isolated. Analysis of the ^{13}C n.m.r. spectrum of the biosynthesized product, and in particular the ^{13}C-^{13}C couplings in ring A of the isoflavonoid, showed that the acetate units were disposed as shown [4.30a]. Hence, cyclization of the putative polyketide intermediate must have occurred via pathway 'a' and not 'b' (Scheme 4.8).

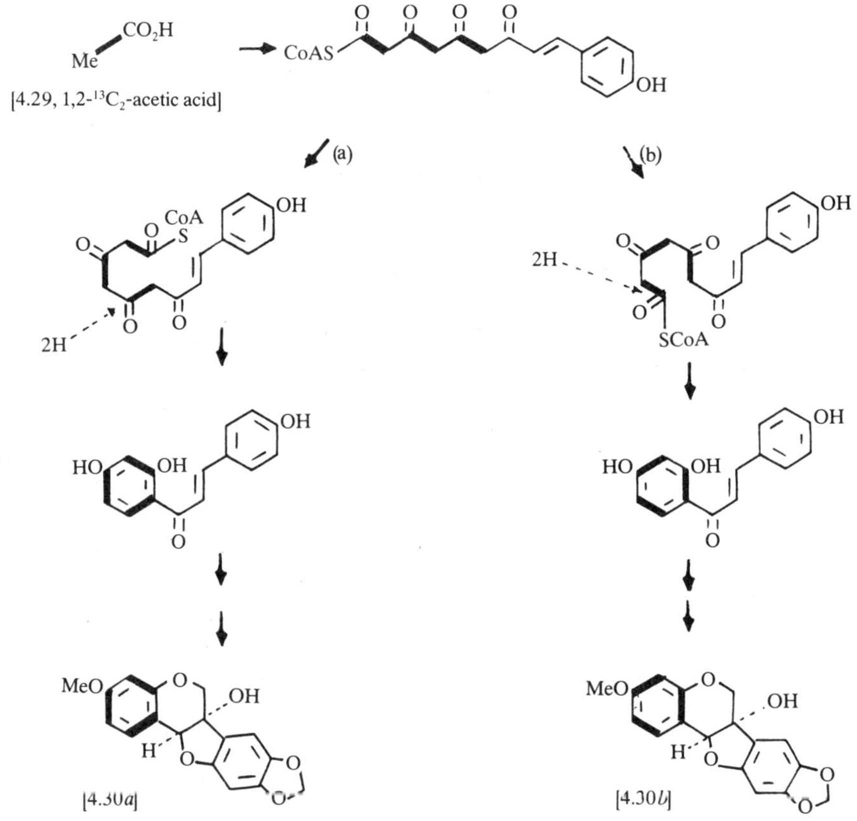

Scheme 4.8. Biosynthesis of pisatin [4.30] from 1,2-$^{13}C_2$-acetate.[21]

References

1. RIBERAU-GAYON, P. *Plant phenolics*. Oliver & Boyd, Edinburgh (1972). HARBORNE, J. B. *Biochemistry of phenolic compounds*. Academic Press, London and New York (1964).

2. HARBORNE, J. B. and CORNER, J. J. *Biochem. J.* **81**, 242 (1961).

3. SWAIN, T. and WILLIAMS, C. A. *Phytochemistry* **9**, 2115 (1970).

4. KOKOUL, J. and CONN, E. E. *J. biol. Chem.* **236**, 2692 (1961).
HAVIR, E. A. and HANSON, K. R. *Biochemistry* **7**, 1896, 1904 (1968).
The biochemistry of plants, Vol. 7 (ed. E. E. Conn), p. 577. Academic Press, London and New York (1981).
HODGKINS, D. S. *J. biol. Chem* **246**, 2977 (1971).

5. NEISH, A. C. *Phytochemistry* **1**, 1 (1961).
HAVIR, E. A., REID, P. D., and MARSH, H. V. *Pl. Physiol.* **48** 130 (1971); ibid. **49**, 480 (1972).

6. NEISH, A. C., in *Biochemistry of phenolic compounds* (ed. J. B. Harborne), p. 295. Academic Press, London and New York, (1964).

7. ZENK, M. H. *Rec. Adv. Phytochem.* **12**, 139 (1979).

8. FREUDENBERG, K. *Science* **148**, 595 (1965).
GRISEBACH, H. *The biochemistry of plants*, Vol. 7 (ed. E. E. Conn), p. 457. Academic Press, London and New York (1981).

9. BATE-SMITH, E. C. *J. Linnaen Soc. (Bot.)* **58**, 95 (1962).

10. HASLAM, E. *Fortschr. Chem. Org. Naturstoffe* **41**, 1 (1982).

11. HASLAM, E. *The shikimate pathway*, pp. 186 and 241. Butterworths, London (1974).

12. LEISTNER, E. *Biochemistry of plants*, Vol. 7 (ed. E. E. Conn), p. 403. Academic Press, London and New York (1981).

13. BENTLEY, R. *Biosynthesis*, Specialist Periodical Reports, Chemical Society, London **3**, 181–246 (1975).

14. HAHLBROCK, K. *The biochemistry of plants*, vol. 7 (ed. E. E. Conn), p. 425; Academic Press, London and New York (1981).
EBEL, J. and HAHLBROCK, K. *The flavonoids* (ed. T. Mabry and J. B. Harborne), p. 641. Chapman & Hall, London (1982).

15. BIRCH, A. J. and DONOVAN, F. W. *Aust. J. Chem.* **6**, 360 (1958).
GEISSMAN, T. A. and CROUT, H. G. D. *Organic Chemistry of Secondary plant metabolites*. Freeman-Cooper, San Francisco (1969).

16. ROBINSON, R. *Structural relationships of natural products*. Clarendon Press, Oxford (1955).

17. GRISEBACH, H. *Rec. Adv. Phytochem.* **1**, 379 (1968).

18. HESS, D. *Planta* **60**, 568 (1964).; *Z. PflPhysiol.* **55**, 374 (1966).

19. PELTER, A., BRADSHAW, J., and WARREN, R. F. *Phytochemistry* **10**, 835 (1971).

20. DEWICK, P. M., *The Flavonoids* (ed. T. Mabry and J. B. Harborne), p. 535. Chapman & Hall, London (1982).

21. STOESSL, A. and STOTHERS, J. B. *Z. Naturf.* **34c**, 87 (1979).

5

TERPENES AND STEROIDS

5.1 Introduction

Terpenes, it has been suggested, are the most abundant and widely-distributed natural products found in plants. It now appears probable that some form of terpene can be synthesized by all organisms, and if to the plant products one adds the ubiquitous steroids and those plant and fungal metabolites which contain one or more branched C_5 units within their structures, then the extraordinary diversity of this group of metabolites can be appreciated (Fig. 5.1). Nature's apparent biosynthetic prodigality is once more amply illustrated. Thus, for example, a wide range of mycotoxins is derived from the α-amino-acid, L-tryptophan [5.1]. Many are obtained by the initial substitution of a γ,γ-dimethylallyl group into the amino-acid nucleus (Scheme 5.1).

Several explanations for this profusion and diversity of terpenoid structures have been advanced. One interesting suggestion is that it represents an example of evolution in progress. According to this idea, the terpenoid pathway of biosynthesis provides the most versatile route to compounds capable of transmitting significant information at all levels of biological organization. Whatever the merits of such speculation, there is little doubt that in the plant kingdom and elsewhere many natural products of a terpenoid origin are now believed to play important biological roles. In this sense these functions and properties have most probably been acquired during the course of evolution. There are, for example, numerous instances where the chemical interaction between species is mediated by terpenoid compounds. Thus, monoterpenes act as agents for communication and defence in the insect population.[1] Several have hormonal or regulatory properties, for example, steroidal hormones, vitamins, and the plant growth regulators—abscissic acid and the gibberillins. Fungal terpenoid hormones have also been described. In *Allomyces* sp., sexual reproduction requires fusion between uniflagellate motile 'male' and 'female' gametes. The hormone which facilitates this approach is a bicyclic sesquiterpene diol, sirenin [5.2], which is active in the attraction of the male gametes at concentrations of 10^{-10} g ml^{-1}. Finally, the various prenyl quinones and the carotenoids should be noted as compounds intimately involved in the physical processes of life— electron transport and photosynthesis respectively.

This diversity of terpene structures is nevertheless bound by a common origin; their molecular architecture is constructed according to a regular structural pattern. Detailed biochemical studies have shown that the terpenoid

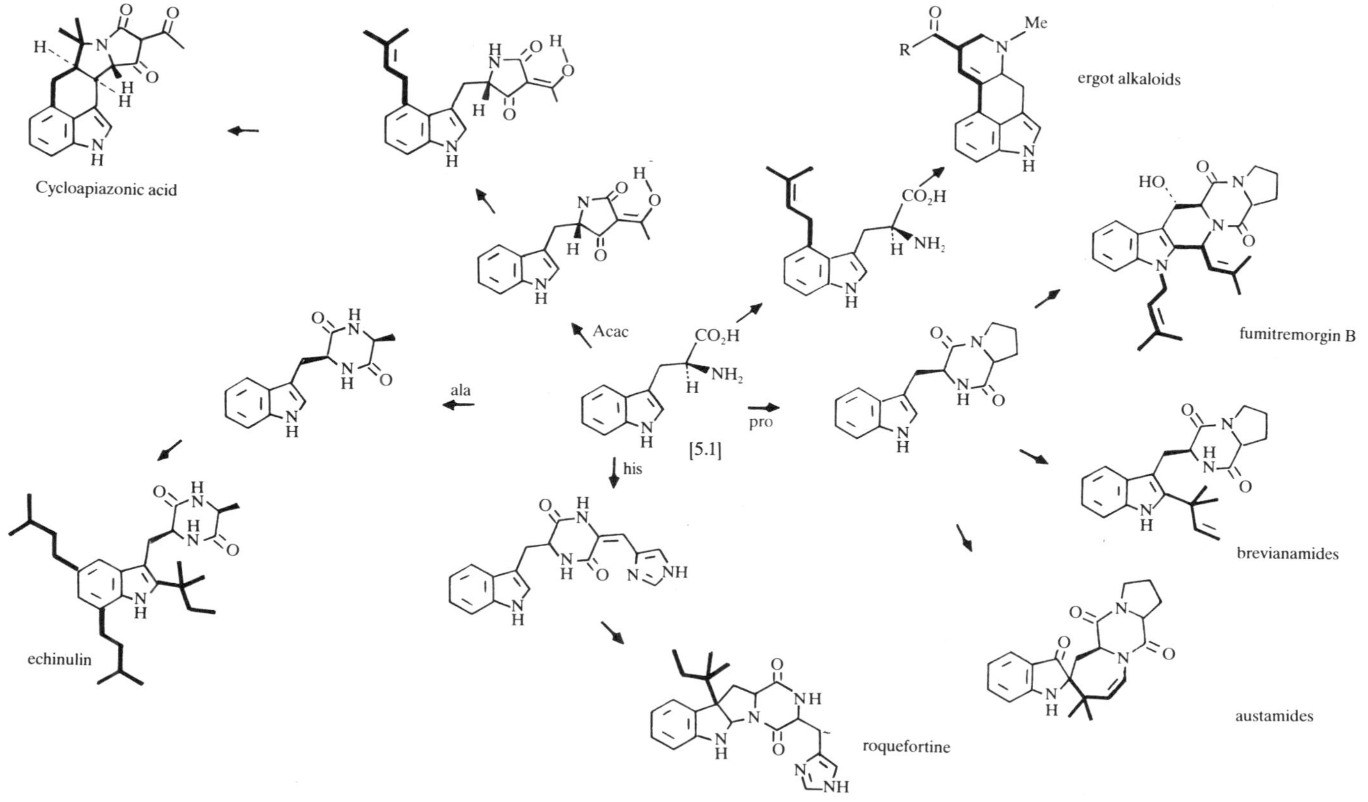

Scheme 5.1. Dimethylallyl-isopentenyl derivatives of tryptophan.

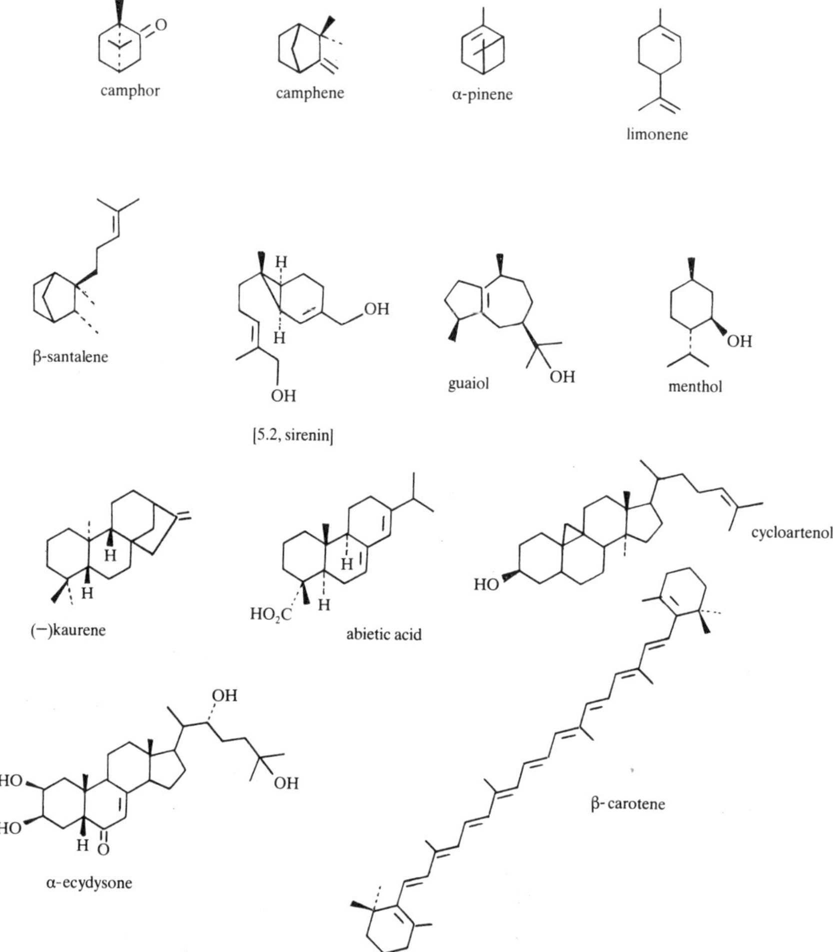

Fig. 5.1. Some terpene and steroid structures.

natural products are synthesized *in vivo* from isopentenyl pyrophosphate ([5.3] IPP) which itself is formed *via* mevalonic acid [5.4] from acetic acid (Scheme 5.2A). (Terpenes are thus related as secondary metabolites to the polyketides). Much of this work has been concerned with mammalian biochemistry and the important sub-group—the steroids. The consensus of observations and views is that, despite occasional anomalies, particularly in plants, these findings form the basis for the understanding of terpene biosynthesis in other organisms.

The art of perfumery, with its connotations of luxury and elegance, was practised by the ancient Chinese and Egyptians and has passed through many stages of development to the exquisite but expensive perfumes of the present day. The new materials of today's perfumes are partly synthetic and partly

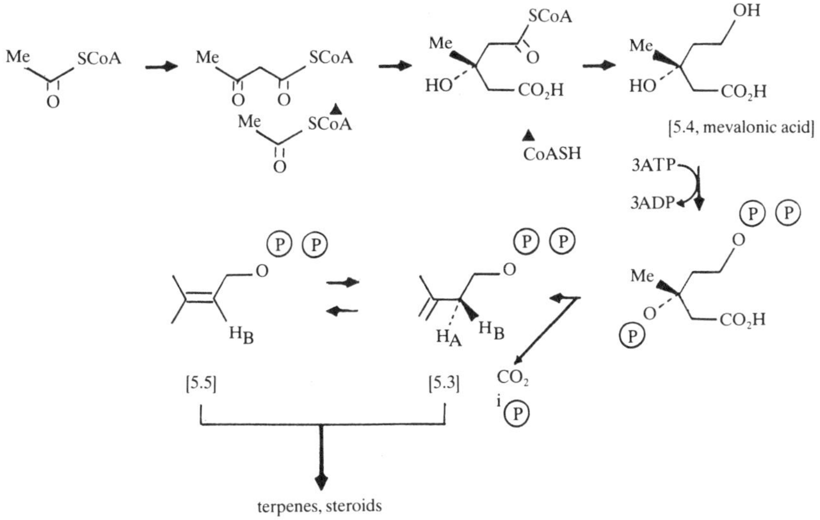

[5.4, mevalonic acid]

[5.5]   [5.3]

terpenes, steroids

[5.3, IPP; isopentenyl pyrophosphate: chain extension unit]
[5.5, DMAPP; dimethylallyl pyrophosphate: chain initiation unit]

Scheme 5.2A. Terpene biosynthesis—the initial steps.

complex mixtures of natural products (essential oils) derived from the leaves, flowers, and fruit of many plants. Typical examples are lavender oil obtained from the flowers of *Lavandula vera*, which has as its major constituents linalool [5.6] and its acetate ester, and rose oil, produced by steam distillation of rose petals, which contain geraniol [5.7] and its dihydro derivative citronellol [5.8].

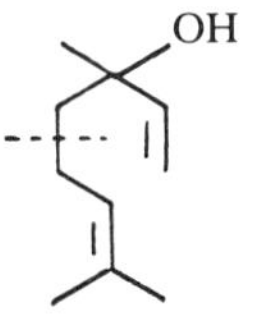

[5.6, linalool] 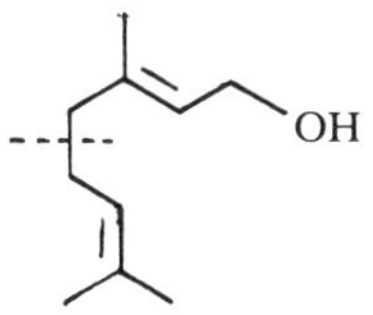   [5.7, geraniol] 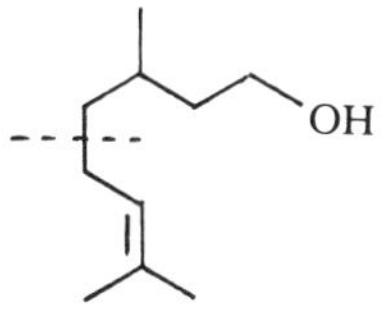   [5.8, citronellol]

The chemistry of these essential oils provided, in every sense of the word, a natural focus for the early practitioners of organic chemistry. The principal component of spirit of turpentine obtained from pine trees is a hydrocarbon pinene $C_{10}H_{16}$ (Fig. 5.1, α-pinene). This same substance occurs in a great many other plants—eucalyptus, juniper, cloves, parsley, sage, thyme, laurel, and lemon. Along with the isomeric hydrocarbons limonene and camphene (Fig. 5.1) it was classified as a terpene. Oxygenated derivatives of the terpenes, such as menthol, camphor (Fig. 5.1), geraniol [5.7], linalool [5.6], and citronellol

[5.8] were also discovered, and the widespread natural occurrence of the mono-terpenes ($C_{10}H_{16}$) and their derivatives, the sesquiterpenes ($C_{15}H_{24}$), the diterpenes ($C_{20}H_{32}$), and triterpenes ($C_{30}H_{48}$), was thus established.

Although Wallach suggested in 1887 that isoprene (C_5H_8) was the funda-mental building unit of the terpenes, the isoprene rule has its antecedents.[29] Thus, Tilden demonstrated that isoprene [5.9] was formed when various cyclic monoterpenes hydrocarbons were thermally decomposed. The inverse observa-tion that dipentene [5.10] (later shown to be the racemic form of limonene) was produced by heating isoprene to 280° was made in 1878 by Bouchardat. This dimerization (one of the earliest examples of the Diels–Alder reaction) exempli-fies the presentiments of the isoprene rule, and these were hinted at by Tilden shortly afterwards.

[5.9, isoprene]   [5.10, dipentene]

Surprisingly, the idea that terpenes were, in principle, structurally composed of isoprene units was not utilized as an acceptable working hypothesis until much later. Thus the structures of α-santalene and farnesol [5.11] were estab-lished in the period 1910–13, both structures are in accordance with the iso-prene rule, yet in neither case was this pointed out.[2] Likewise, Willstätter, in 1911, advanced a structure for the terpenoid alcohol phytol which was not in agreement with the empirical rule.[2]

[5.11, farnesol]

5.2 The isoprene rule and the biosynthesis of terpenes

The subsequent establishment of the isoprene rule owes a great deal to Ruzicka[2] and the systematic study of the higher terpenes which started in Zurich in the 1920s. The classical isoprene rule has essentially two parts: the first which states that the terpene skeleton is divisible into a regular array of isoprene units, and the second which says that the isoprene units are generally arranged in a 'head-to-tail' (1–4) formation (cf. geraniol, citronellol, linalool, farnesol, *vide supra*). The fundamental steps in normal terpene biosynthesis which lead to this 1–4 or 'head-to-tail' linkage of isoprene units are shown in Schemes 5.2A and 5.2B. Δ^3-Isopentenylpyrophosophate [5.3] is isomerized by an enzymically-controlled 1,3-allylic shift to give 3,3-dimethylallyl pyrophosphate [5.5]. Chain elongation proceeds by adding isopentenyl pyrophosphate ([5.3] IPP) initially to 3,3-dimethylallyl pyrophosphate ([5.5] DMAPP) to give geranyl pyrophosphate [5.12]. The reaction pathway, represented formally in Scheme 5.2B, probably involves a two-step mechanism involving an enzyme-bound intermediate and proceeds with clearly defined stereochemistry at the three participating centres.[3] The geranyl pyrophosphate ([5.12] C_{10}) then functions as the allylic partner in the next condensation step to yield farnesyl pyrophosphate ([5.13] C_{15}), and geranylgeranyl pyrophosphate ([5.14] C_{20}) is generated by adding a further C_5 (IPP) unit.

Like all empirical rules, the isoprene rule does not lay down an infallible law, and as the knowledge of terpene chemistry expanded then so did the exceptions to the dogma. The hydrocarbons squalene [5.15] and phytoene [5.26] thus contain two isoprene units linked in irregular 'tail-to-tail' (4–4) fashion. Other compounds, although clearly derived from isoprene units, such as lavandulol [5.17], artemisia ketone [5.18], and chrysanthemic acid [5.19], could not be accommodated within the same simple rule.[2]

'Tail-to-tail' (4–4) linkage of isoprene units has subsequently been shown to occur by a quite different and rather complex mechanism.[4] It occurs in the generation of the hydrocarbon squalene from two molecules of farnesyl pyrophosphate (Scheme 5.3), and a similar reaction is probably involved in the formation of phytoene [5.16] by the dimerization of geranylgeranyl pyrophosphate [5.14]. In the production of squalene, an intermediate with a three-membered ring—presqualene pyrophosphate [5.20]—is formed, and this is then reductively cleared to give squalene, (Scheme 5.3).

It has been suggested, in this particular context, that the small but very interesting group of irregular monoterpenes (e.g. artemisia ketone and lavandulol, *vide supra*) are formed by ring cleavage of trans-chrysanthemyl alcohol (the C_{10} analogue of presqualene and prephytoene alcohols) (Scheme 5.4). Recently, trans-chrysanthemyl alcohol [5.21] has been found to be a natural product in its own right, and cell-free extracts of *Artemisia* and *Santolina* species converted both *cis*- and *trans*-chrysanthemyl alcohols into artemisia ketone. In the formal classical sense, all these reactions may be envisaged as occurring from the carbocation [5.22] or its enzyme-bound equivalent.

5.3 The biogenetic isoprene rule

In 1937, the elucidation of the structure of eremophilone [5.25] caused something of a sensation.[2] It was the first sesquiterpene with a carbon skeleton that could not formally be subdivided into isoprene units. Robinson proposed that

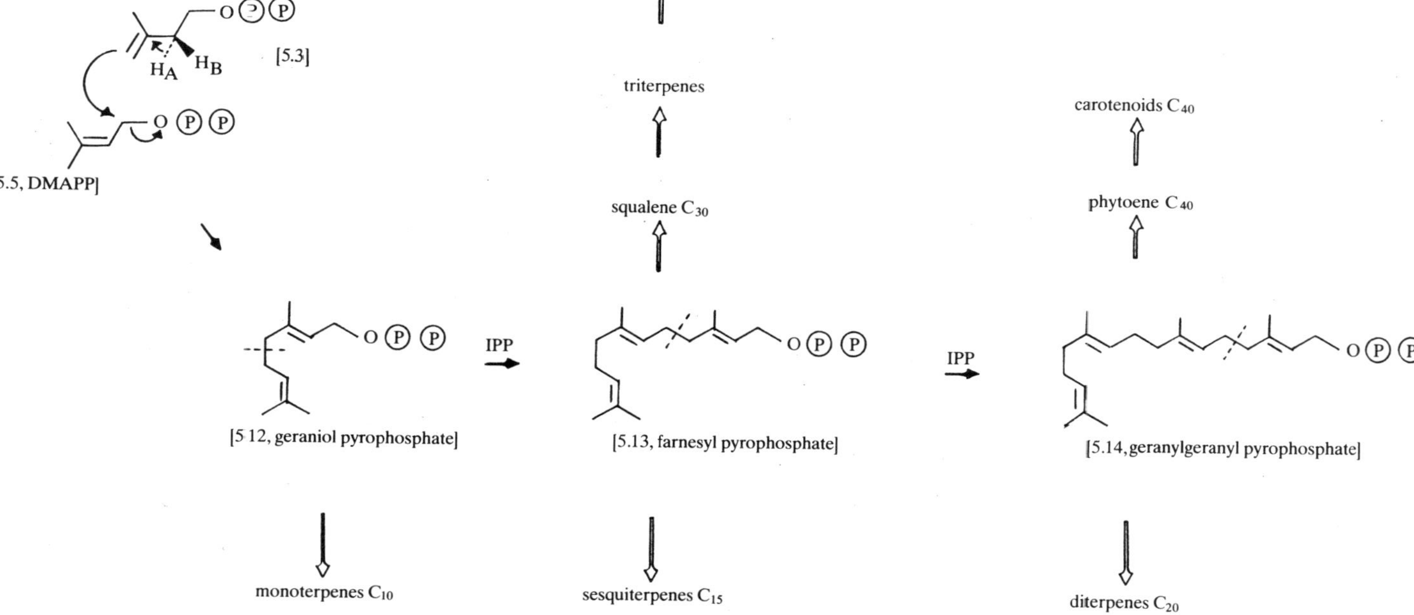

Scheme 5.2B. Biosynthesis of terpenes, steroids, and carotenoids.[3]

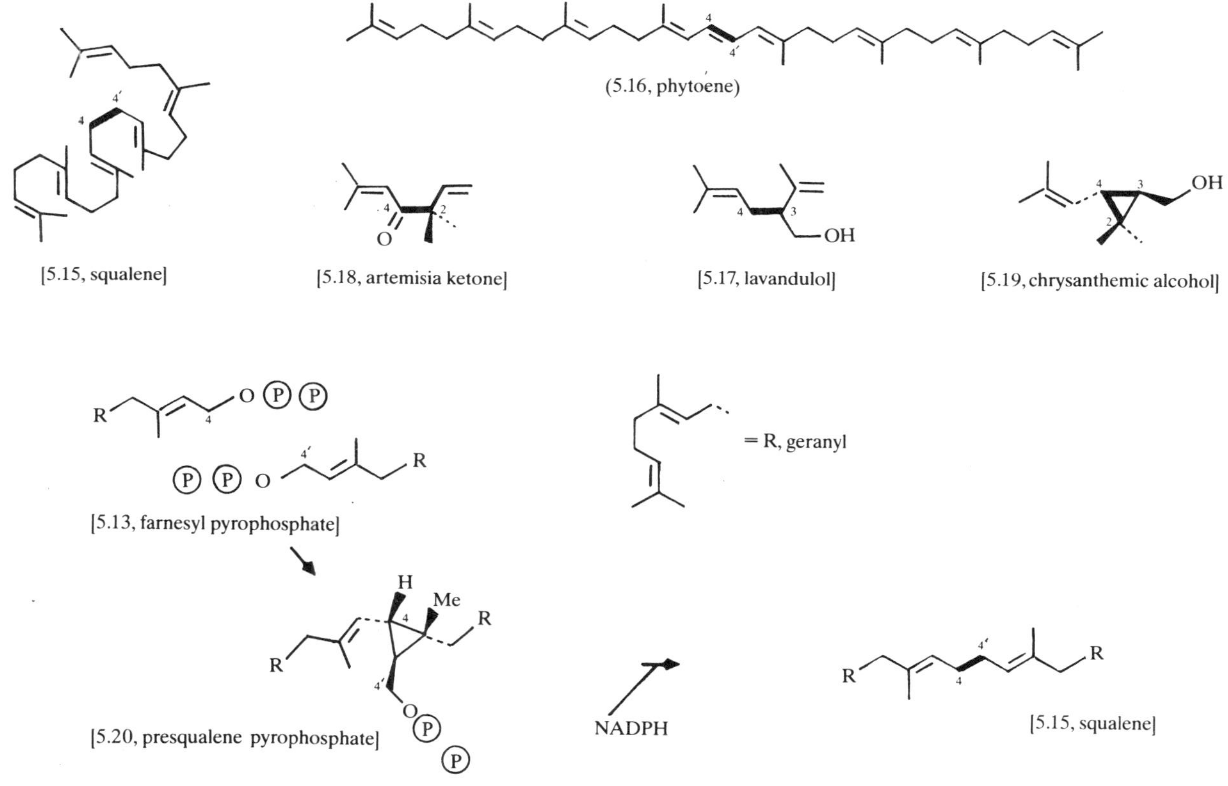

Scheme 5.3. Biosynthesis of squalene.[4]

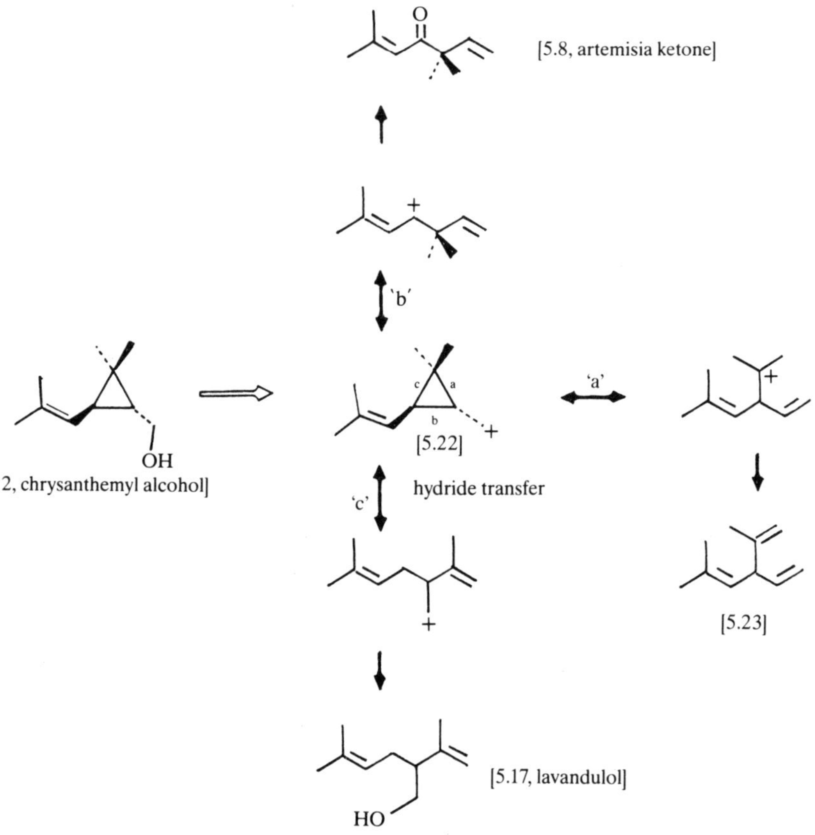

[5.8, artemisia ketone]

'b'

[5.12, chrysanthemyl alcohol]

[5.22]

'a'

hydride transfer

'c'

[5.23]

[5.17, lavandulol]

Scheme 5.4. Proposed biosynthesis of irregular monoterpenes.[5]

this structure might originate by rearrangement accompanying dehydration of a hypothetical precursor [5.24] of the eudesmol type. Robinson's suggestion[6] was a harbinger of much that was to follow, and in particular of the unifying and perspicacious biogenetic isoprene rule devised by Ruzicka.[2]

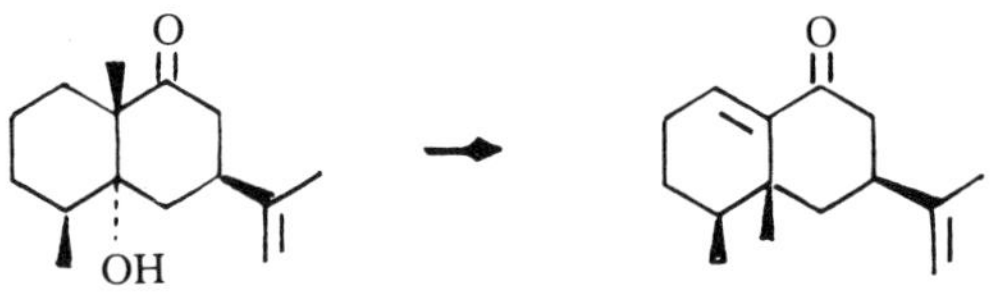

[5.24]

[5.25, eremophilone]

The evolution of this hypothesis is intimately linked with the development of the story of the biosynthesis of cholesterol.[3,4,7] There had been much speculative thinking upon this exceptionally challenging problem. In 1926,

Shannon had shown[7] that squalene [5.15] fed to animals increased the cholesterol content of the tissues, and, once the structure of cholesterol [5.27] had been proven, Robinson[1] indicated in the early 1930s that the carbon skeleton of the sterol might be derived by cyclization of the hydrocarbon squalene. In 1952, the structure of lanosterol [5.26] was finally settled; it was important for several reasons. It contradicted the classical isoprene rule, and it led Woodward and Bloch to argue incisively that it could be derived by cyclization of squalene and formation of a carbocation intermediate with subsequent migration of two hydrogen atoms and two methyl groups. The proposals had an immediate appeal. They uniquely rationalized the structure of lanosterol [5.26], and by inference placed it on the pathway to cholesterol from squalene.

Subsequent experimentation has substantiated this view.[7] The oxidative cyclization of squalene is chemically one of Nature's most remarkable biosynthetic reactions. It is a two-stage process, and involves 2,3-oxidosqualene [5.28] as an intermediate. Although the reaction (Scheme 5.5) is characterized by a very high degree of stereospecificity, it is believed that the primary role of the enzyme (apart from acting as a proton donor) is to impose a specified conformation on the substrate. Once this has been attained the cyclization sequence may simply be regarded as an exploitation of the inherent chemical reactivity of the substrate molecule.

In higher plants and algae, the initial sterol formed from 2,3-oxidosqualene [5.28] is not lanosterol but cycloartenol [5.29]. Basically, the reaction may be formulated in a similar way, but in this instance the 9β-H is postulated to migrate to C-8, and the C-9 carbonium ion is captured from the α-face by a nucleophilic group on the enzyme surface. A 1,3-anti-elimination of a proton from the C-19 methyl group and the nucleophile would then lead to cycloartenol [5.29] (Scheme 5.6).

Contemporaneously with the unfolding of the squalene–cholesterol story, the idea that the regular acyclic terpenes geranyl pyrophosphate [5.12], farnesyl pyrophosphate [5.13] and geranylgeranyl pyrophosphate [5.14], could by dimerization and/or cyclization and rearrangement act as precursors to all of the various sub-classes of terpenes (Scheme 5.2B) was a view developed by Ruzicka.[2] The concept is enshrined in the *biogenetic isoprene rule*.

Ruzicka's ideas,[2] and the subsequent experimental work on the biosynthesis of terpenes, once again powerfully exemplify the precept that Nature obeys the laws of chemistry: in this case it is the chemistry of carbocations. However, it should be borne in mind that the representation in these schemes of intermediates as carbocations is merely a convenient symbolism, and the formulation of reaction pathways with carbocation species is a purely formal device. The actual species are not known; they may be pyrophosphate esters or enzyme-bound equivalents of carbocations. In most cases it is the acyclic olefin rather than an oxiran derivative (as with squalene, *vide supra*) which is envisaged as the substrate for cyclization. As with squalene, however, it is stereoelectronic

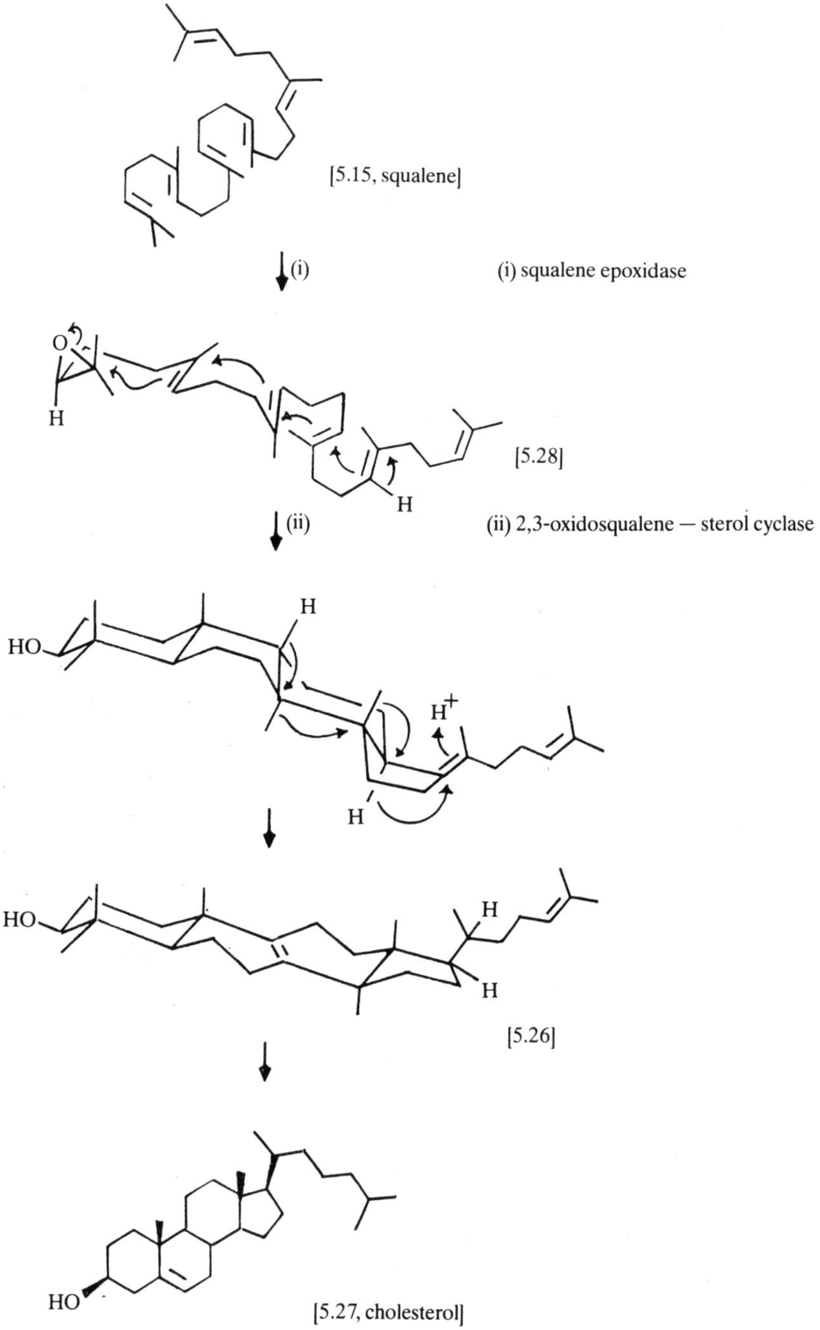

Scheme 5.5. Biosynthesis of cholesterol from squalene.[7]

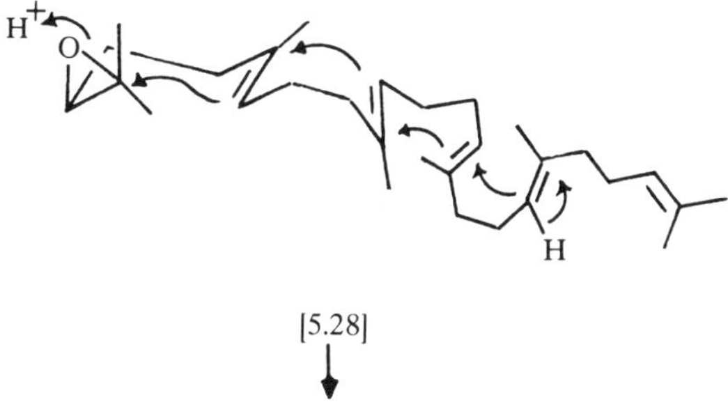

Scheme 5.6. Biosynthesis of cycloartenol.[8]

factors inherent in the substrate molecule itself which profoundly influence the biosynthetic pathways developed. The cyclization reactions themselves may be formulated in differing ways. Either as:

(i) initial protonation of a double bond;

bisabolene

or (ii) initial nucleophilic attack of a double bond on the pyrophosphate ester group or the same reaction formulated in terms of the equivalent carbocation species.

neryl pyrophosphate

In the sesquiterpene and diterpene class reactions of this type are believed to occur, giving macrocylic compounds which may then undergo further cyclizations or rearrangements:

5.3.1 Monoterpenes (C_{10})

Monoterpenes are derived from geranyl pyrophosphate (Schemes 5.2 and 5.7). For steric reasons cyclization to the various mono- and bicyclic derivatives occurs via its 2-cis-diastereoisomer neryl pyrophosphate (or the equivalent carbocation).

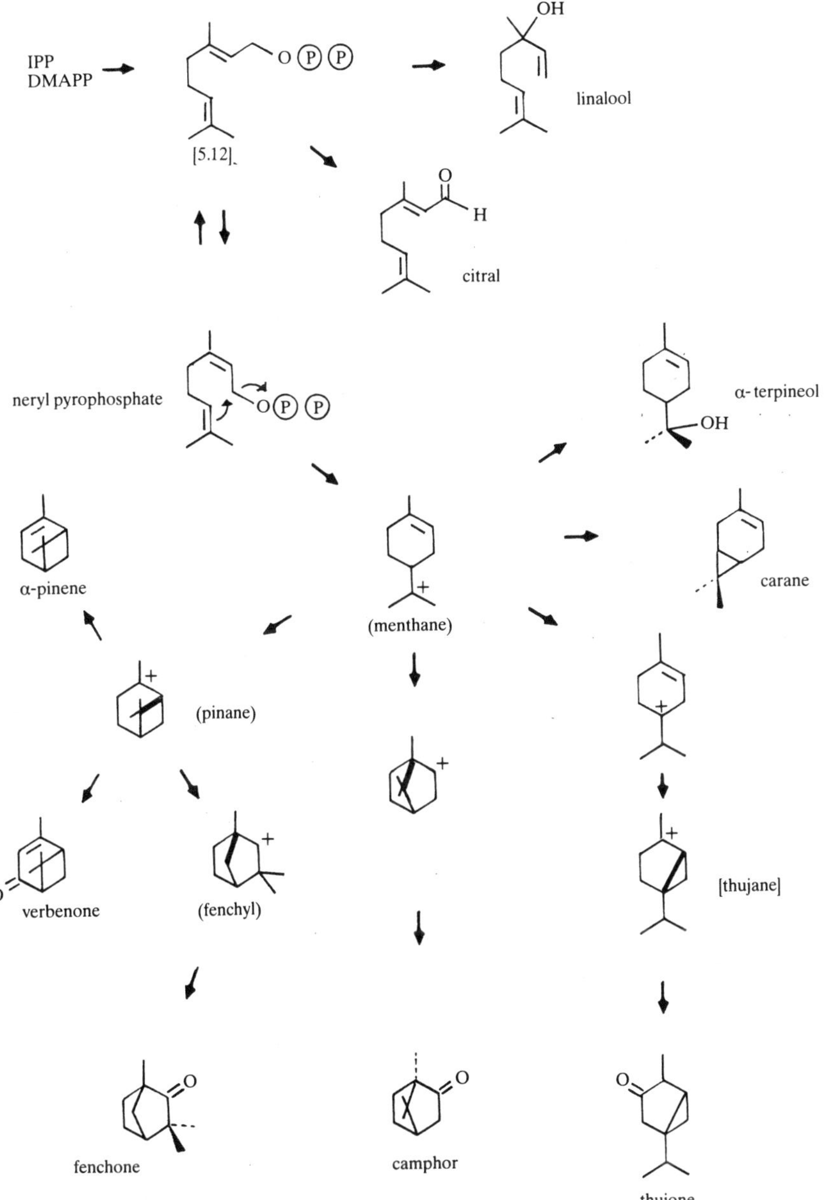

Scheme 5.7. Biogenetic isoprene rule: cyclic monoterpenes.

The carbon skeletons once formed are then functionalized (oxidation, reduction, etc.) by relatively unspecific enzymes acting within a metabolic grid. Tracer studies have broadly confirmed the correctness of Ruzicka's views,[2] although often in plants only that portion of the molecule derived from isopentenyl pyrophosphate (IPP [5.3]) is significantly labelled by isotopic tracer. Some correction is necessary to the view of the way in which the carane skeleton is developed. Feeding of 2-[14]-C-mevalono-lactone [5.30] to *Pinus* sp. resulted in a labelling pattern for (+)-car-3-ene as shown [5.31]. This suggested that the second cyclization occurs with double-bond migration.

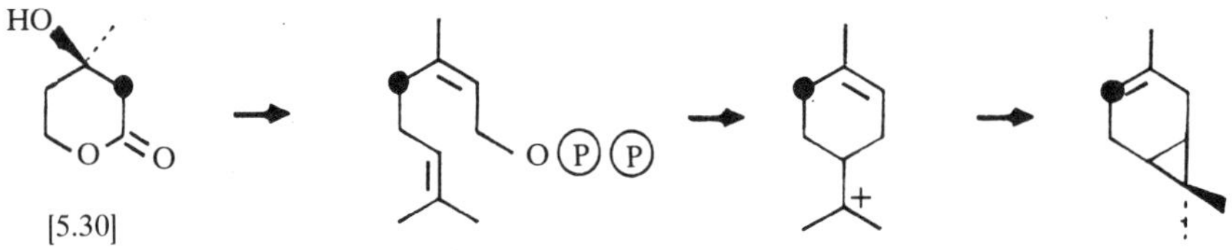

[5.30]

[5.31]

$\bullet$ = ^{14}C

5.3.2 Sesquiterpenes (C$_{15}$)

From the biogenetic viewpoint, Nature has been extraordinarily prolific in the synthesis of sesquiterpenes.[9] Indeed, they probably exhibit a greater structural and stereochemical diversity than any other class of terpene. Ruzicka's biogenetic speculation has been extensively documented, although detailed experimental verification of many of the proposals is still awaited.

According to the biogenetic proposals, either 2-cis- or 2-trans-farnesyl pyrophosphate ([5.32] or [5.13]) undergoes transformation to the various carbocations [5.33]–[5.38] by the processes described above. Almost all the known sesquiterpene types can then be derived from these ions by wholly rational chemical steps. Some examples best illustrate the concepts involved (Schemes 5.9–5.16).

In the case of 2-cis-farnesyl pyrophosphate [5.32], interaction of the allylic pyrophosphate (or carbocation) with the central olefinic linkage leads to the monocylic cations [5.33], [5.34]. Many of the known six-membered monocyclic sesquiterpenes, such as bisabolene [5.39] and γ-curcumene [5.40], can be derived from the carbocation [5.33]. Protonation of the terminal double bond of γ-bisabolene [5.39] followed by cyclization then leads to the bicyclic systems [5.41] and [5.42]. Alternatively, an electronically-favoured stereospecific cyclization of bisabolene furnishes the carbocation [5.43], the logical precursor of sesquiterpenes such as cedrol [5.44] (Scheme 5.9).

Analogously, oxidative modification of the carbocation [5.35] generates all the ten-membered ring sesquiterpenes with the germacrane skeleton such as germacrone [5.45] (Scheme 5.10). Trans-annular cyclization of the carbocation

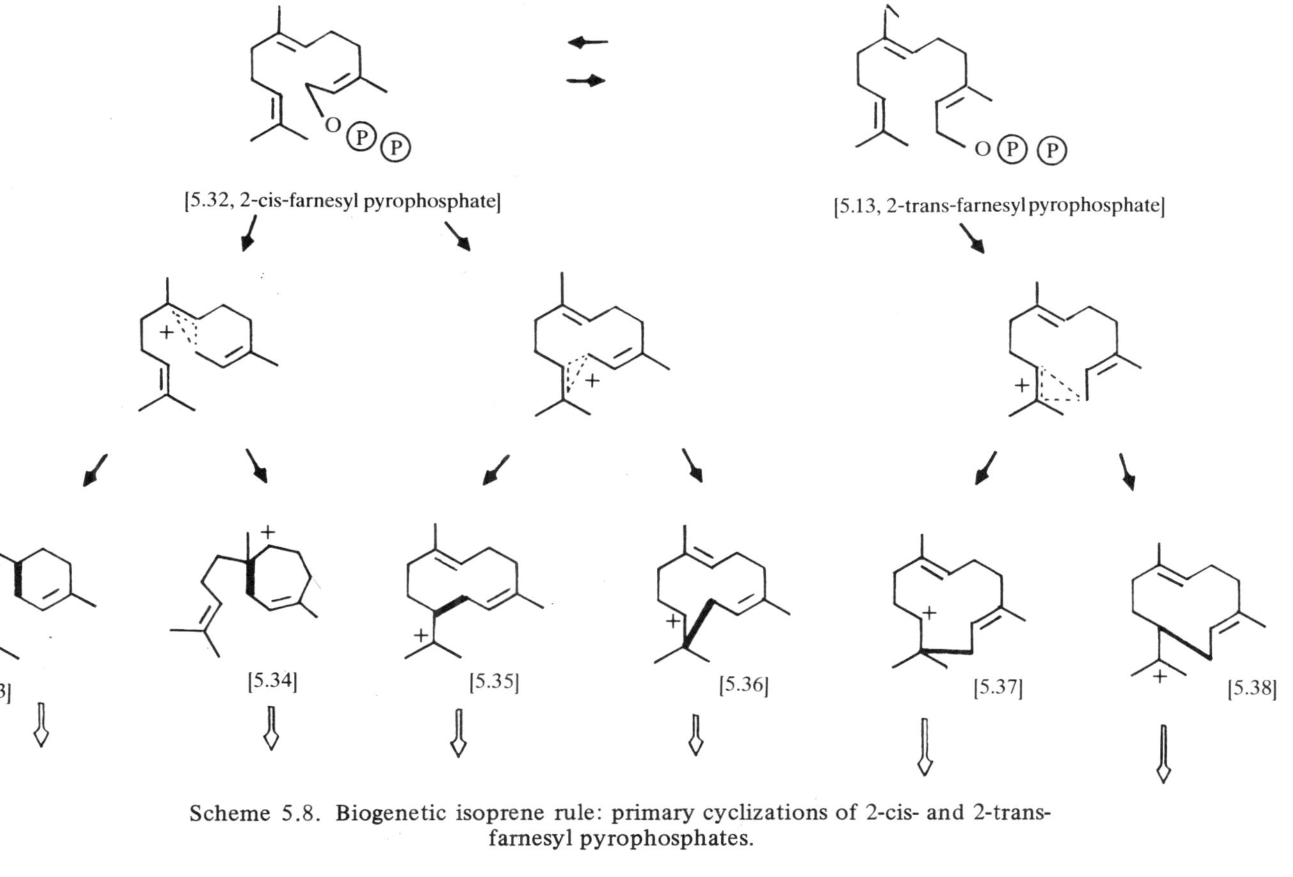

Scheme 5.8. Biogenetic isoprene rule: primary cyclizations of 2-cis- and 2-trans-farnesyl pyrophosphates.

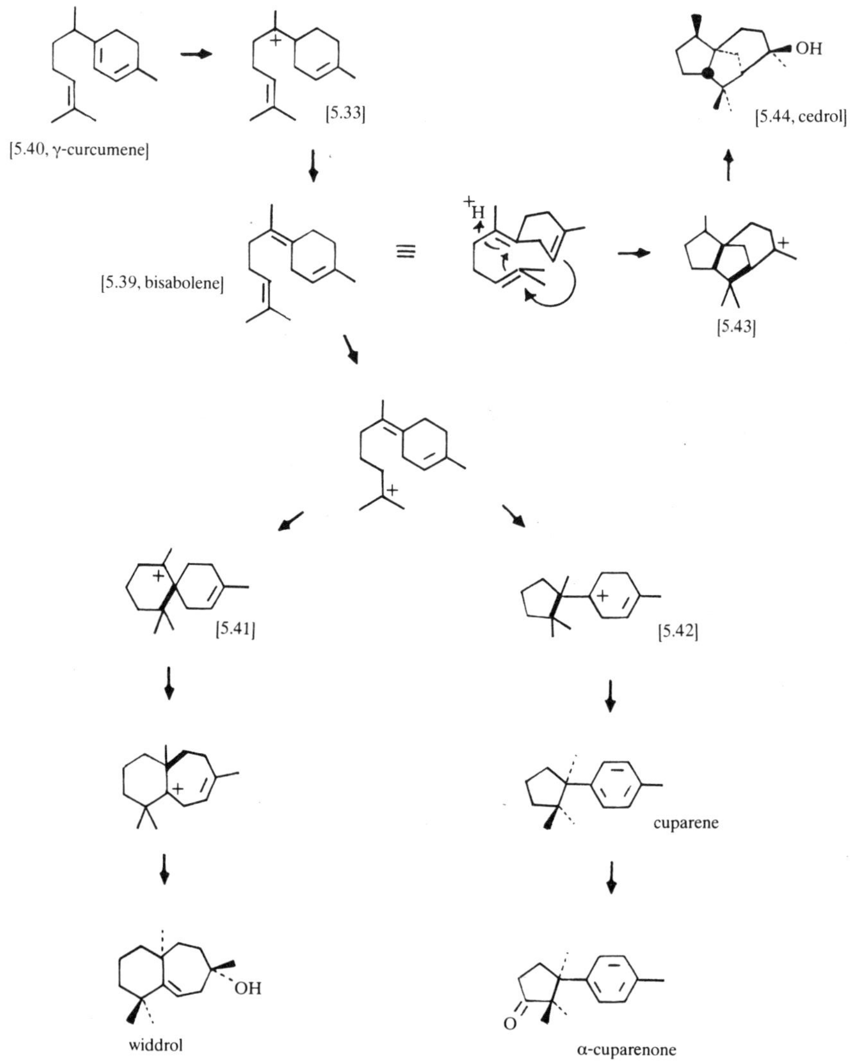

[5.40, γ-curcumene]

[5.33]

[5.39, bisabolene]

[5.44, cedrol]

[5.43]

[5.41]

[5.42]

cuparene

widdrol

α-cuparenone

Scheme 5.9. Sesquiterpene biogenesis.

[5.35], or a derivative, in the Markownikoff fashion, gives the eudesmane series [5.46]. Anti-Markownikoff cyclization of the same cation (or derivative) generates the guaiane skeleton [5.47].

Although detailed experimental verification of many of these speculative schemes is still awaited, there has recently been a substantial volume of experimentation in this area.[5] In several cases this provides elegant proof of these ideas.

[5.45, germacrone]

[5.35]

H$_3$O$^+$ H$_3$O$^+$

[5.46, α-eudesmol]   [5.47, guaiol]

Scheme 5.10. Sesquiterpene biogenesis.

Overton[10] has thus studied the generation of γ-bisabolene [5.39] and the oxidatively-derived metabolite paniculide B [5.48] in callus cultures of *Andrographis paniculata*. That 2-cis, 6-trans-farnesyl pyrophosphate, [5.32], (and not the 2-cis, 6-cis isomer), is the biosynthetic precursor of γ-bisabolene [5.39] was established by incorporation (1.2 per cent) of 3R- 2-^{14}C, 5-^{3}H$_2$-mevalonic acid [5.49] (Scheme 5.11), into the hydrocarbon with loss of one-sixth of the tritium label. This supports the intermediacy of the 2-cis, 6-trans isomer [5.32] itself derived from the 2-trans, 6-trans isomer with loss of a hydrogen atom ($\frac{1}{6}$th loss of ^{3}H) from the terminal methylene group in the inter-conversion. Paniculide B [5.48], biosynthesized from 1,2-^{13}C$_2$-acetate, was shown to retain 'intact' acetate units located in the carbon skeleton as indicated, and this is quite consistent with the above speculations and conclusions (Scheme 5.11).

One sesquiterpene-derived metabolite whose biosynthesis has been examined[11] in some depth is avocettin [5.50] in *Anthostoma avocetta*. The original concept of its derivation was that it was formed by oxidative degradation of (−)-γ-cadinene (Scheme 5.12). Three different mechanistic pathways can, in principle, be delineated from the farnesyl precursor [5.13] to (−)-γ-cadinene and hence avocettin [5.50] (Scheme 5.12). Incorporation (0.12 per cent) of 2-trans-6-[^{3}H]-farnesyl pyrophosphate [5.13] into avocettin [5.50], with retention of the isotope in the predicted position, was proved by base-catalysed conversion of the metabolized avocettin [5.50] to [5.51], when greater than 80 per cent loss of the tritium was observed. Further proof was furnished by the incorporation of 2-^{14}C-mevalonolactone [5.52] into avocettin. This showed the origin

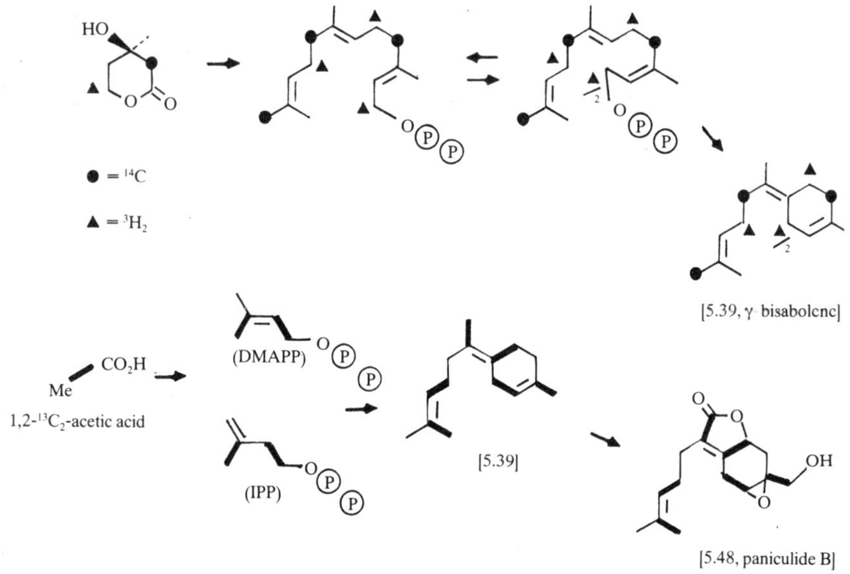

Scheme 5.11. Biosynthesis of γ-bisabolene and paniculide B: sesquiterpene biogenesis.[10]

of the critical carbon atoms in the carbon framework of the metabolite, and demonstrated the particular folding [5.13a] adopted by the 2-trans-farnesyl pyrophosphate precursor (Scheme 5.13).

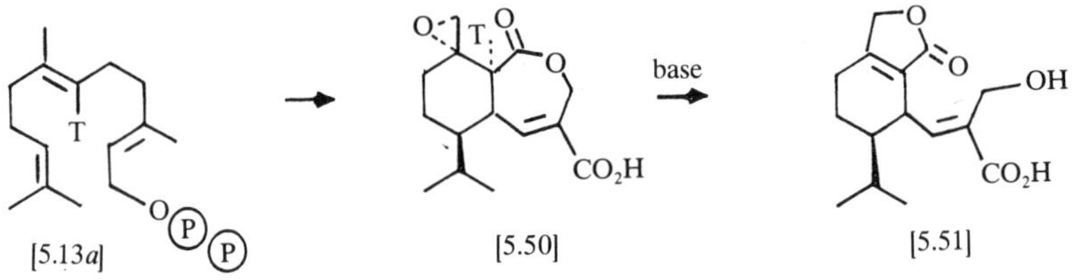

Confirmation of this view, and of the role of all trans-farnesyl pyrophosphate [5.13] as the first C_{15}-intermediate on the biosynthetic pathway to avocettin, was obtained using 4R-[³H]-mevalonic acid lactone [5.53] as precursor. Knowledge of the metabolism of mevalonic acid to isopentenyl pyrophosphate [5.3] and dimethylallyl pyrophosphate [5.5] leads to the prediction that one tritium atom equivalent will be located in each of the three double bonds of [5.13], and this will lead, as was found, to location of the isotope at the predicted positions in avocettin [5.50] (Scheme 5.14).

Evidence, finally, as to the detailed mechanistic pathway adopted in the conversion of all trans-farnesyl pyrophosphate [5.13] to (−)-γ-cadinene and hence avocettin [5.50] was derived from the results of the incorporation of

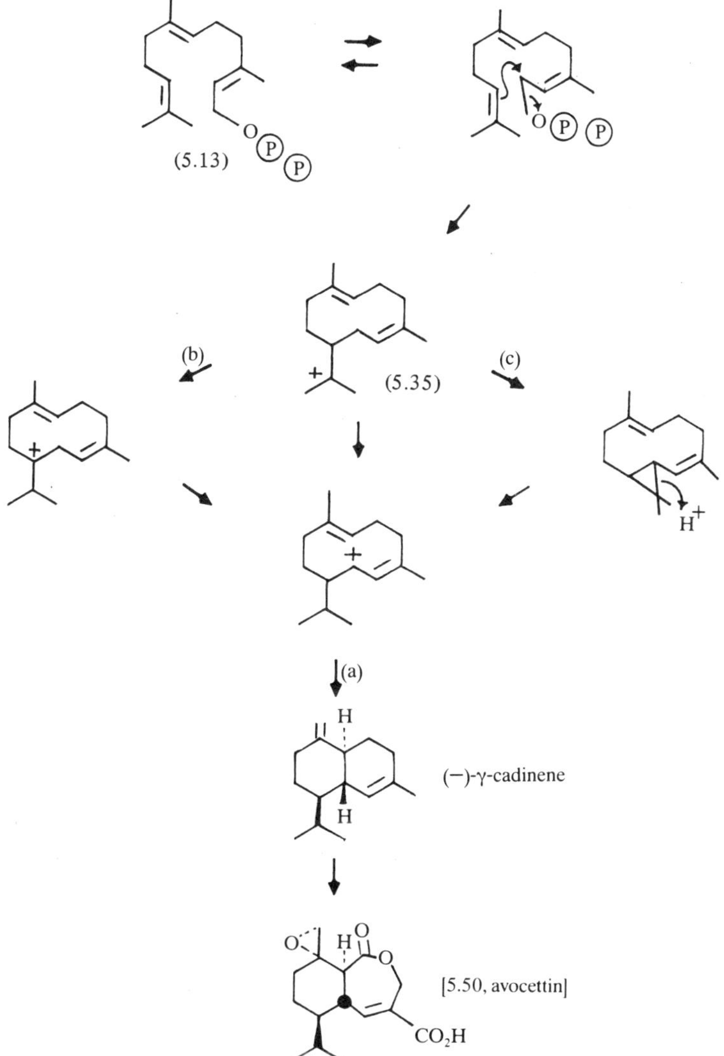

Scheme 5.12. Possible biosynthetic pathways to avocettin.[11]

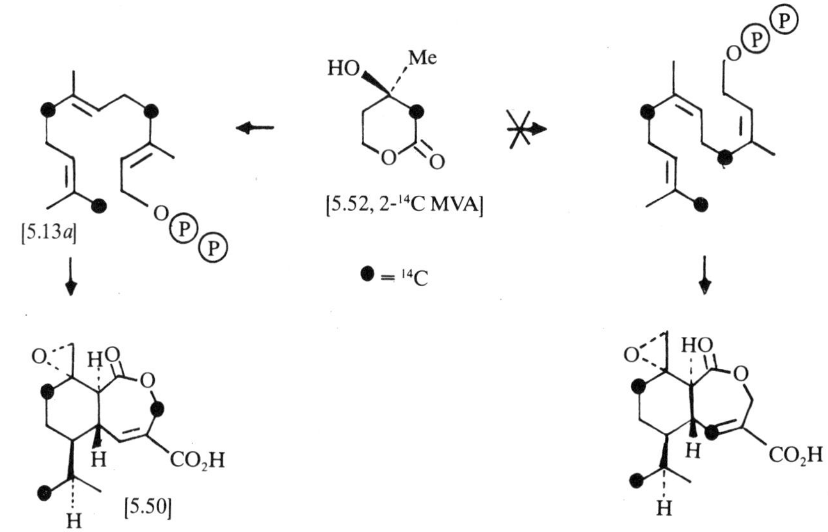

Scheme 5.13. Biosynthesis of avocettin: folding of the farnesyl chain.[11]

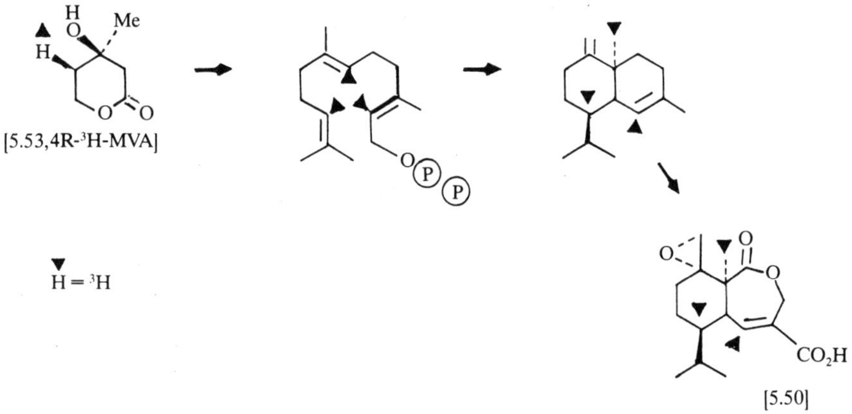

Scheme 5.14. Biosynthesis of avocettin from 4R-[^{3}H]-mevalonolactone.[11]

5R-[^{3}H]-and 5S-[^{3}H]-labelled mevalonolactones as precursors [5.54a,b] (Scheme 5.15). These results demonstrate that no loss of H occurs from the terminal methylene group of farnesyl pyrophosphate and that saturation of the isopropyl side-chain occurs *via* a 1,3-hydride shift (route 'a', Scheme 5.12). Moreover, this 1,3-hydride shift occurs specifically by transfer of H_B. These observations lead to the formulation of the biosynthetic pathway to avocettin [5.50] as shown (Scheme 5.16) *via* the hydrocarbon germacrene D [5.55].

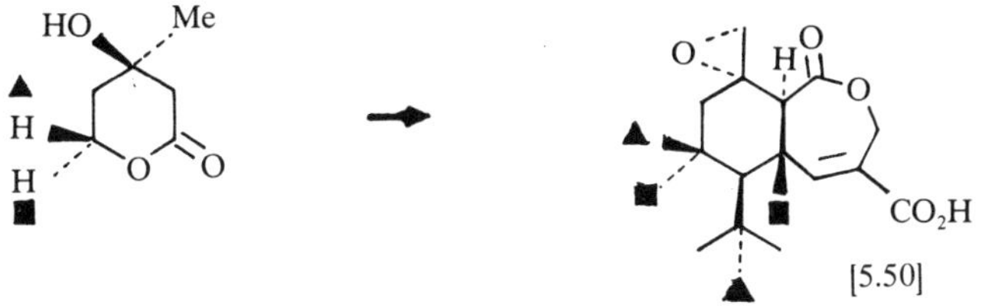

[5.50]

[5.54a, 5R-³H]; ■ = ³H

[5.54b, 5S-³H]; ▲ = ³H

Scheme 5.15. Biosynthesis of avocettin from 5R- and 5S-[³H]-mevalonolactone.[11]

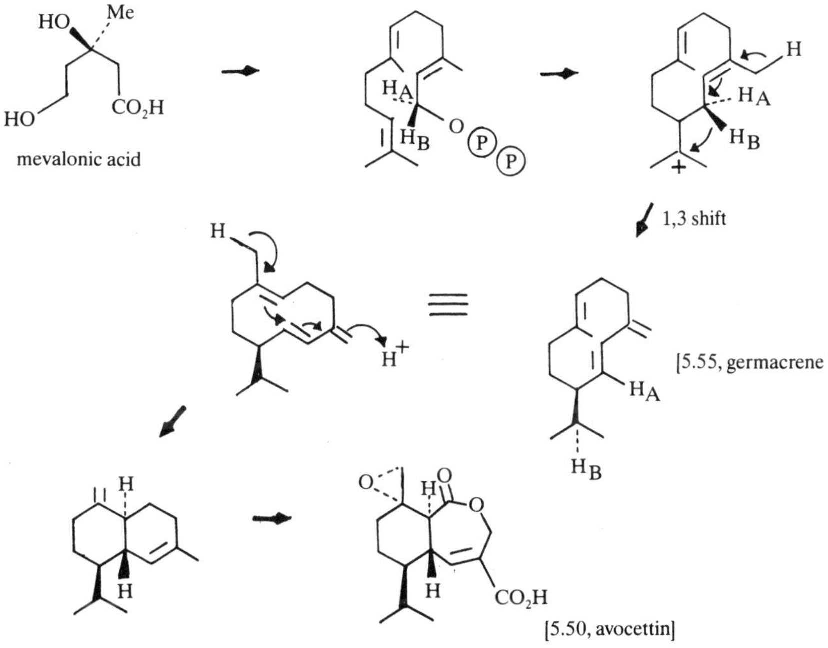

mevalonic acid

1,3 shift

[5.55, germacrene D]

[5.50, avocettin]

Scheme 5.16. Biosynthesis of avocettin (Arigoni[11]).

5.3.3 Diterpenes (C_{20})

Diterpenes are invariably considered[12] to be formed from geranylgeranyl pyrophosphate [5.14]. Most diterpenes are cyclic and possess no hydroxyl group at C-3, and the implication is that such compounds appear to be formed by a simulated stereospecific direct acid-catalysed cyclization of the substrate [5.14]. This reaction may be formally represented as a proton-initiated sequence commencing at the distal isoprene unit. Hypothetical biogenetic routes from

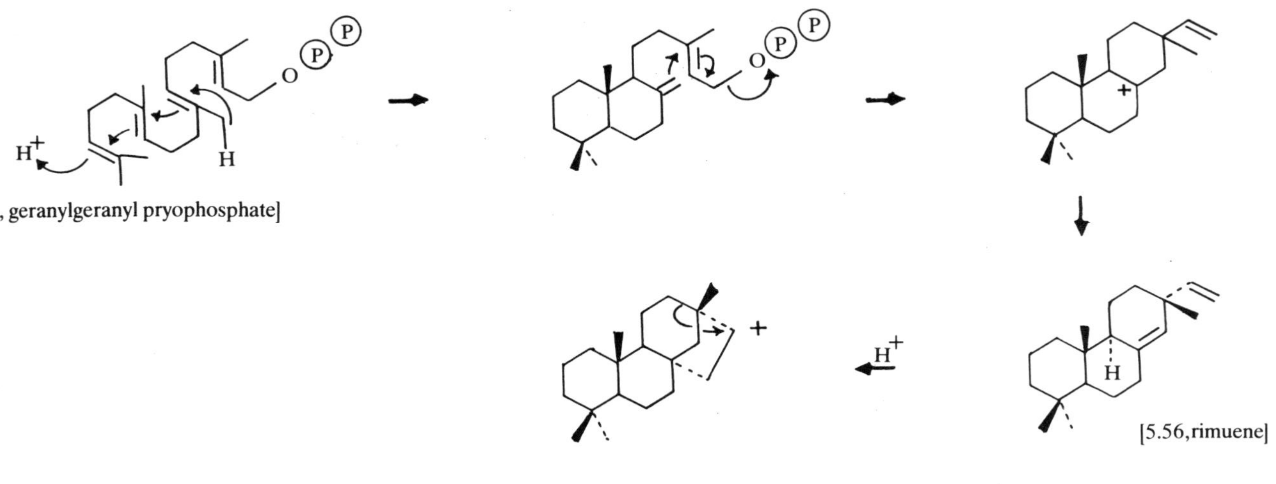

Scheme 5.17. Diterpene biogenesis.[12]

[5.14] to most of the classes of diterpenes have been proposed, e.g. rimuene [5.56], abietic acid [5.57], and phyllocladene [5.58].

The gibberellins[13] are a group of diterpenoid substances which are recognized as having great importance in the regulation of plant growth.[14] They were first discovered, however, through an investigation of a plant disease, the 'foolish seedling' disease of rice in the Orient. This disease is characterized by the astonishing growth of rice seedlings which, however, subsequently never reach maturity. Examination of the abnormality showed that it was caused by a fungus *Gibberella fujikuroi* and a metabolite which was named gibberellin. The first physiologically-active compound to be isolated and identified was gibberellic acid or GA_3: well over fifty gibberellins are now described in the literature. Gibberellins occur in most if not all green plants, and they possess important regulatory functions. Responses of plants to exogenously-applied gibberellins indicates that the effects produced are those normally controlled by phytochrome or induced by chilling. The most accessible gibberellin, GA_3 [5.59] is used commercially in horticultural practice.

The diterpenoid origin of the gibberellins was established by Birch who found that $2\text{-}^{14}\text{C}$-mevalonolactone and $1\text{-}^{14}\text{C}$ acetate were incorporated into GA_3 [5.59] by cultures of *Gibberella fujikuroi* with a labelling pattern consistent with this derivation. The first step in the biosynthetic pathway to the gibberellins was elucidated using cell-free enzyme extracts of the seed *Echinocystis macrocarpa* in the presence of ATP. It was demonstrated that mevalonolactone was converted to geranylgeranyl pyrophosphate [5.14] via geranyl and farnesyl pyrophosphate. In the presence of Mg^{2+}, this system facilitated the cyclization of [5.14] to the hydrocarbon (−)-entkaurene [5.61] and later work indicated that copalyl pyrophosphate [5.60] was an intermediate in this sequence. (−)-Entkaurene [5.61] is the parent hydrocarbon of the gibberellins and it illustrates one of the distinctive features of diterpene biosynthesis—namely, the formation of ring junctions which are antipodal to the normal (steroid-like) found in other diterpene substances such as abietic acid [5.57]. The constant absolute stereochemistry which is observed in the triterpenes is not maintained in the diterpenes.

The next stage in the biosynthesis involves the stepwise oxidation of the C-19 methyl group of (−)-entkaurene [5.61] to a carboxyl function and hydroxylation of ring B. Ent-7-α-hydroxykaurenoic acid [5.62] is a substrate for the characteristic ring contraction in gibberellin metabolism (*, Scheme 5.18), which then leads ultimately to compounds such as GA_3 [5.59] by loss of the angular C-20 methyl group (Scheme 5.18).

5.3.4 Triterpenes (C_{30})

The brilliant demonstration[7] that squalene, via its 2,3-epoxide [5.28], is the precursor of lanosterol [5.26], and hence cholesterol [5.27] (Scheme 5.5),

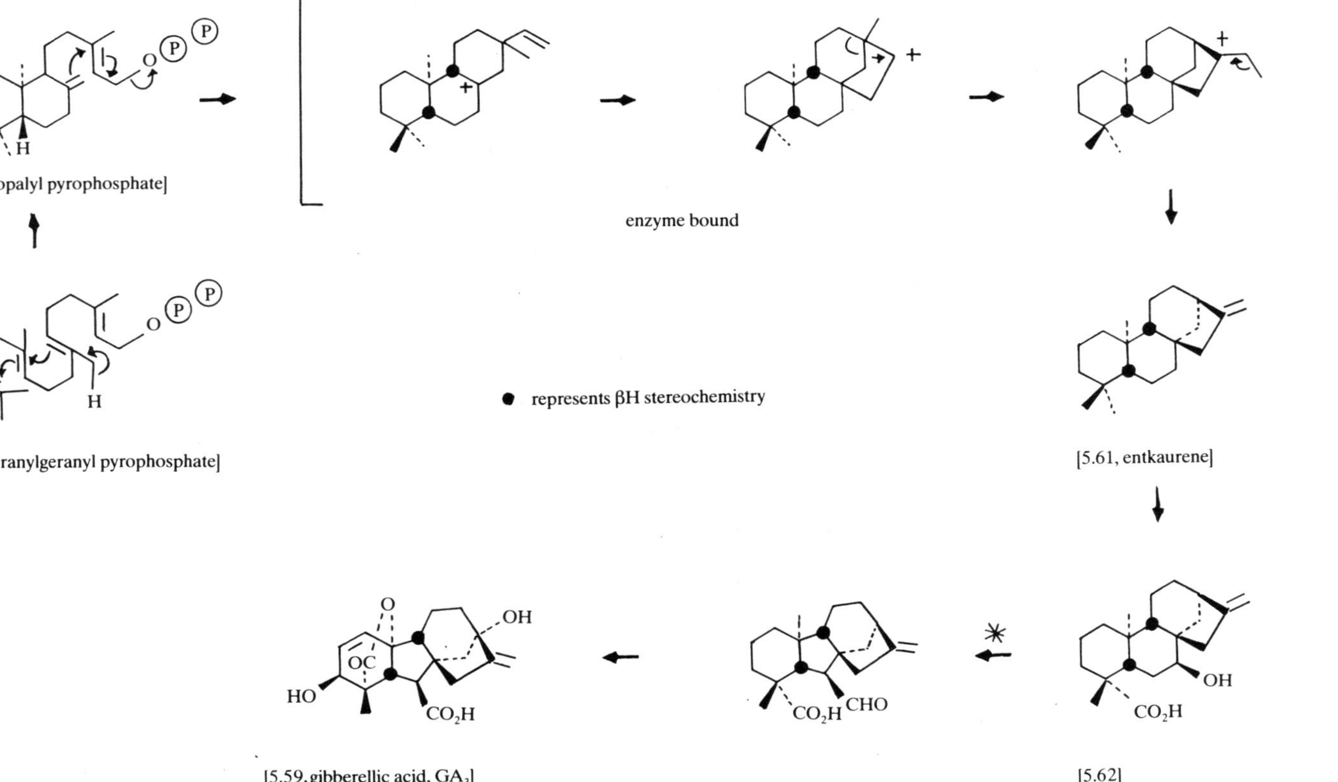

Scheme 5.18. Biosynthesis of gibberellic acid.[13]

and its rationalization in terms of a concerted series of stereoelectronically-controlled cyclizations was quickly followed[15] by elegant proposals for the derivation of non-steroidal triterpenes from the same acyclic hydrocarbon. Various rules, based on chemical precedent, were formulated. Chief amongst these were:

> (i) for each cyclization step the squalene molecule is folded (on the enzyme surface) in a series of potential chair-like or boat-like six-membered rings;
>
> (ii) the cyclizations proceed by a concerted sequence of planar *trans* additions to the olefinic double bonds;
>
> (iii) discharge of the intermediate carbocation may follow Wagner–Meerwein rearrangements and hydride shifts if the optimal stereo-electronic circumstances appertain.

The proposals are both elegant and impressive and enable a whole series of triterpenoid structures to be rationalized under one biosynthetic umbrella. Thus, folding of squalene epoxide in the chair-chair-chair-boat-unfolded conformation, leads *via* a concerted, proton-initiated, cyclization to the intermediate [5.63] (Scheme 5.19). Its capture leads to tetracyclic triterpenes such as damarenediol [5.64]. The entry into the pentacyclic triterpenes (e.g. germanicol and lupeol) is achieved by cyclization of the same conformation of squalene, but with the intervention of a 'pause' for rearrangement after the generation of the intermediate [5.63] (Scheme 5.19).

Confirmation that S-squalene-2,3-epoxide is a precursor of the pentacyclic triterpenes, such as depicted in Scheme 5.19, has been obtained using pea seedlings.[16] Delineation of some of the steps involved in the rearrangement of the postulated intermediate carbocation [5.63] has been derived[16] using tissue cultures of *Isodon japonicus*. Thus, administration of 4-^{13}C-mevalonic acid [5.66] gave the metabolite oleanic acid [5.65] containing six carbon atoms enriched with ^{13}C isotope. The pattern of labelling in rings D and E confirmed the biogenetic pathway outlined (Scheme 5.19). Similarly, administration of 4R-4-^{3}H-2-^{14}C-mevalonic acid [5.67] gave the metabolite labelled with tritium in ring E as predicted (Scheme 5.20), from the discharge of the carbocation via a β-armyrin type structure.

5.4 Biomimetic polyene cyclizations

When, in 1955, Eschenmoser and Stork pointed out that the biological cyclization of squalene-2,3-epoxide could be rationalized on stereoelectronic grounds their hypothesis stimulated a whole range of biomimetic studies.[17] Although early attempts to imitate *in vitro* polyene cyclizations were not promising, later work has led to biogenetic-type syntheses of several complex polycyclic triterpenoids which closely parallel the biosynthetic pathways themselves. Various

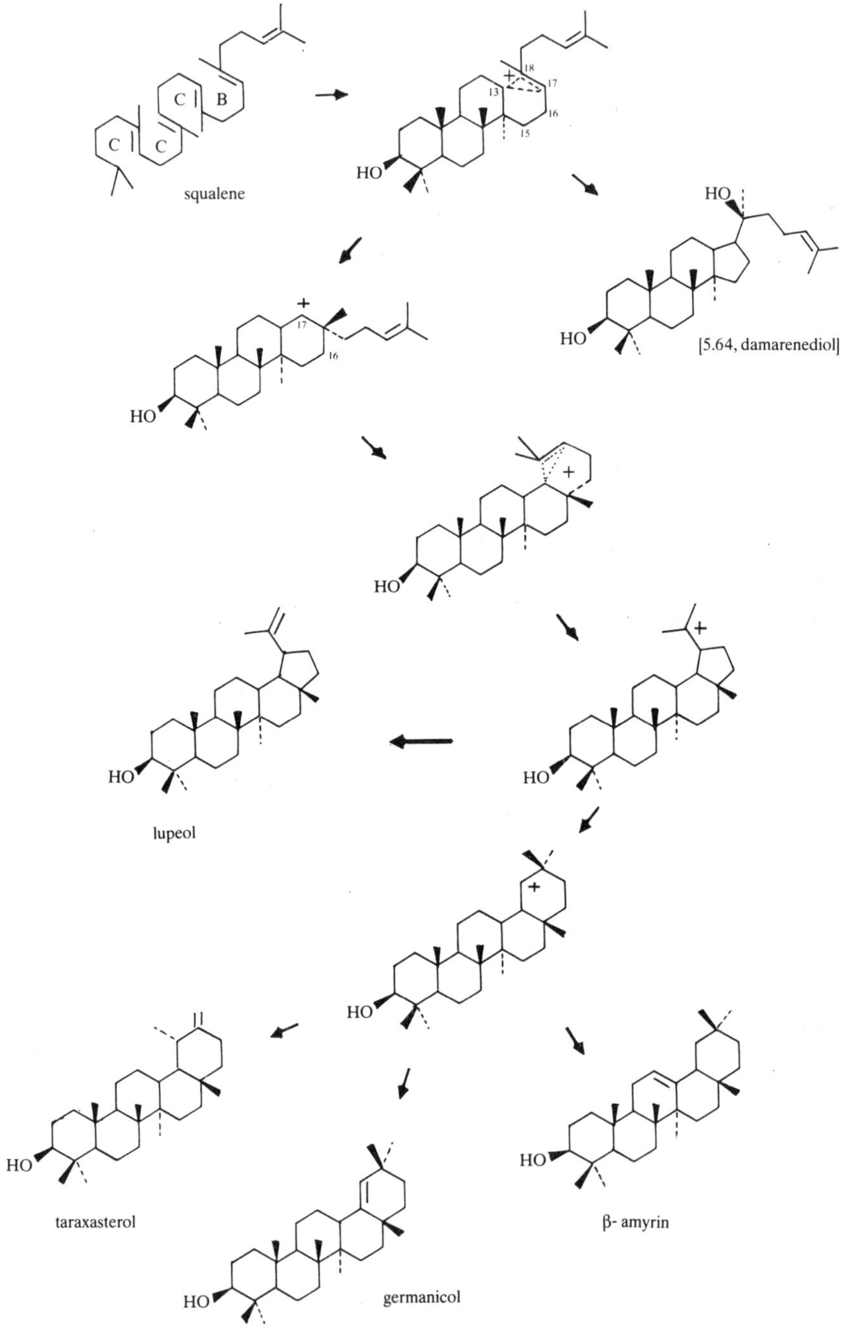

Scheme 5.19. Biogenetic pathways to some triterpenes.[15]

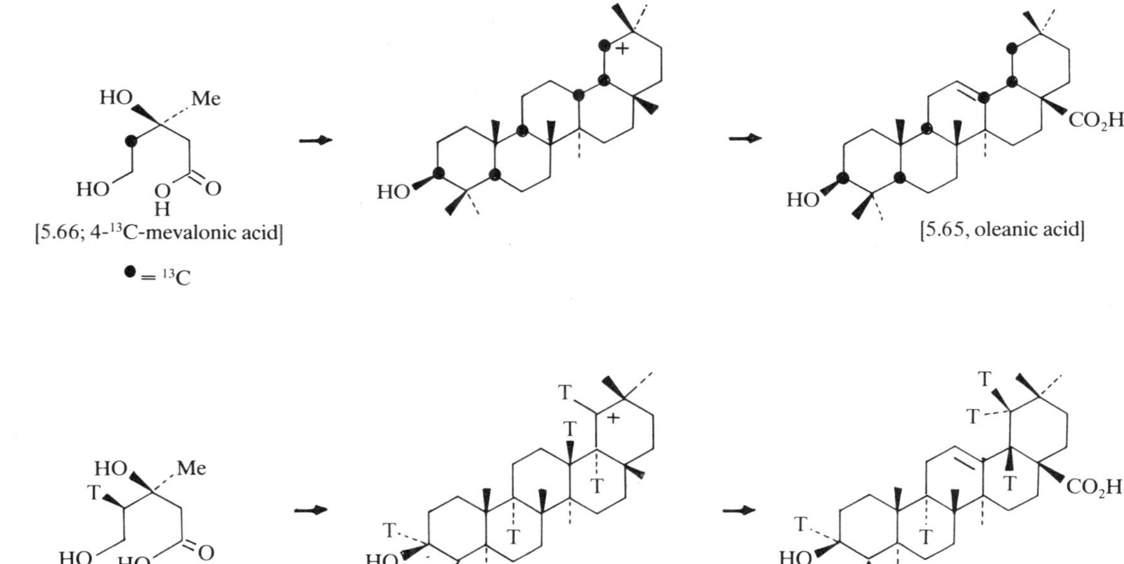

Scheme 5.20. Biosynthesis of oleanic acid in *Isodon japanicus*.[16]

studies have concentrated on the different methods most suitable for the generation of a cationic centre on carbon to initiate polyene cyclization. Van-
Tamelen[17-19] has examined the potential of protonation of a terminal epoxy
function to set up the cyclization sequence. As such, this work directly models
the enzymic system(s) which act on substrates such as squalene-2,3-epoxide.

Using this approach, for example, a successful synthesis of pentanorisoeuphenol
[5.69] was accomplished by treatment of the epoxide [5.68] with $SnCl_4$ in
nitromethane to give a 35 per cent yield of the alcohol.[18]

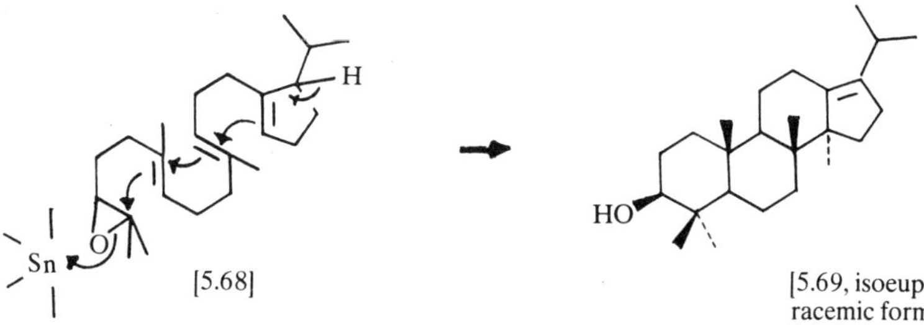

[5.68]

[5.69, isoeuphenol]
racemic form

In an extension of this work, the epoxide [5.70] similarly treated responded
to give $(\pm)$-δ-amyrin ([5.71] 8 per cent). Resolution via the (S)-methoxytri-
fluoromethylphenyl acetate derivative gave the natural $(-)$-δ-amyrin [5.71].

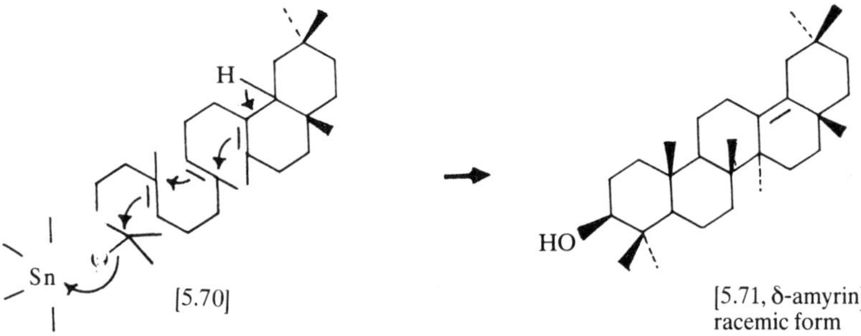

[5.70]

[5.71, δ-amyrin]
racemic form

References

1. HARBORNE, J. B. *Introduction to ecological biochemistry*. Academic
   Press, London and New York (1977).
   BU'LOCK, J. D. in *The filamentous fungi*, Vol. 2 (ed. J. E. Smith and
   D. R. Berry). Edward Arnold, London (1976).
2. RUZICKA, L. *Proc. Chem. Soc.* 341 (1959).
   RUZICKA, L. *Experentia* **9**, 357 (1953).
   RUZICKA, L. *A. Rev. Biochem.* **42** 1 (1970).

RUZICKA, L. *J. pure & appl. Chem.* **6**, 493 (1963).

3. POPJAK, G. and CORNFORTH, J. W. *Biochem. J.* **101**, 553 (1966).
   CORNFORTH, J. W. *Chem. Soc. Rev.* **2**, 1 (1973).
   CORNFORTH, J. W., CORNFORTH, R. H., DONNIGER, C., and POPJAK, G. *Proc. Roy. Soc.* **B163**, 492 (1966).
   ARCHER, B. L., BARNARD, D., COCKBAIN, E. G., CORNFORTH, J. W., CORNFORTH, R. H., and POPJAK, G. *Proc. Roy. Soc.* **B163**, 519 (1966).
   CORNFORTH, J. W. *Chem. Br.* **6**, 431 (1970).

4. CORNFORTH, J. W. *Chem. Soc. Rev.* **2**, 1 (1973).
   EPSTEIN, W. W. and RILLING, H. C. *J. biol. Chem.* **245**, 4597 (1970).
   EDMOND, J., POPJAK, G., WONG, S.-M., and WILLIAMS, V. P. *J. biol. Chem.* **246**, 6254 (1971).
   BEYTIA, E., QUARESHI, A. A., and PORTER, J. W. *J. biol. Chem.* **248**, 1856 (1979).
   POULTER, C. D. and RILLING, H. *Acc. Chem. Res.* **11**, 307 (1978).

5. BANTHORPE, D. V., and CHARLWOOD, B. V. *Secondary plant products —Encyclopedia of plant physiology*, Vol. 8 (ed. E. A. Bell and B. V. Charlwood), p. 185. Springer-Verlag, Heidelberg and New York (1980).
   BATES, R. B. and PANIKER, S. K. *Tetrahedron Lett.* 1453 (1965).
   SHAW, J., NOBLE, T., and EPSTEIN, W. *J. Chem. Soc., Chem. Commun.* 590 (1975).

6. ROBINSON, R. *Structural relationships of natural products.* Clarendon Press, Oxford (1955).

7. SABINE, J. R. *Cholesterol.* Marcel Dekker, New York (1977).
   BLOCH, K. *Science* **150**, 19 (1965).
   SHANNON, H. J. *Biochem. J.* **20**, 400 (1926).

8. WALSH, C. *Enzymatic reaction mechanisms.* Freeman, San Francisco (1979).

9. RUCKER, G. *Angew. Chem. int. edn.* **12**, 793 (1973).
   PARKER, W., ROBERTS, J. S., and RAMAGE, R. *Qt. Rev. Chem. Soc.*, **21**, 331 (1967).

10. OVERTON, K. H. and PICKEN, D. J. *J. Chem. Soc., Chem. Commun.* 105 (1976).

11. ARIGONI, D. *J. pure & appl. Chem.* **41**, 219 (1975).

12. HANSON, J. R. in *Comprehensive organic chemistry*, Vol. 5 (ed. E. Haslam). Pergamon Press, Oxford (1979).

13. MACMILLAN, J., HEDDEN, P., and PHINNEY, M. *A. Rev. Pl. Physiol.* **29**, 149 (1978).
    HANSON, J. R. *Fortschr. Chem. Org. Naturstoffe* **29**, 395 (1978).
    RAILTON, I. D. *S. African J. Sci.*, **72**, 371 (1976).
    WEST, C. A. in *Biosynthesis and its control in plants* (ed. B. V. Millborrow), p. 143. Academic Press, London and New York (1973).

14. GALSTON, A. W. and DAVIES, P. J. *Control mechanisms in plant development.* Prentice-Hall, New Jersey (1970).

15. ESCHENMOSER, A., RUZICKA, L., JEGER, O., and ARIGONI, D. *Helv. Chim. Acta* **38**, 1890 (1955).
STORK, G. and BURGHSTAHLER, A. W. *J. Am. Chem. Soc.* **77**, 5068 (1955).

16. BARTON, D. H. R., JARMAN, T. R., WATSON, K. G., WIDDOWSON, D. A., BOAR, R. B., and DAMPS, K. *J. Chem. Soc., Chem. Commun.* 861 (1974).
SEO, S., TOMITA, Y., and TORI, K. *J. Chem. Soc., Chem. Commun.* 270 (1975).

17. JOHNSON, W. S. *Bioorganic chemistry* **5**, 51 (1976).
VAN TAMELEN, E. E. *Acc. Chem. Res.* **8**, 152 (1975).

18. VAN TAMELEN, E. E., MILNE, G. M., STUFFNESS, M. I., RUDLER-CHAUVIN, M. C., ANDERSON, R. J., and ACHINI, R. S. *J. Am. Chem. Soc.* **92**, 7202 (1970).

19. VAN TAMELEN, E. E., SEILER, M., and WIERRENGA, W. *J. Am. Chem. Soc.* **94**, 8229 (1972).

6

SOME GENERAL CHARACTERISTICS OF SECONDARY METABOLISM

Earlier in the text the proposition was advanced that the nature and functions of secondary metabolism can only be comprehended properly in terms of the whole metabolic matrix from which it derives. Acceptance of such a proposition necessitates that any discussion of secondary metabolism must therefore be placed in the context of the particular relationship to primary metabolism, its enzymology and control. The task is still in its infancy and a great deal remains to be accomplished before this goal can be achieved. Nevertheless, some of the more general characteristics of secondary metabolism and metabolites have begun to emerge, and these are highlighted in the following discussion.

6.1 Stage of development of organism

One important characteristic of secondary metabolism which has been noted is its frequent dependence on the developmental stage of the organism.[1] Often there is a close correlation between the expression of secondary metabolism and morphological and cytological changes—for example, antibiotic synthesis and sporulation in fungi. Similarly, at the gross microbiological level, many of the industrially-important antibiotic batch fermentations can be divided into distinct phases. Generally, antibiotic accumulation during the exponential phase (tropophase) of growth is negligible, but is maximal in a subsequent phase (idiophase) of relatively high metabolic activity during which vegetative growth is arrested. These phases are especially apparent in the highly-productive mutant organisms, and the factor that controls the onset of antibiotic biosynthesis is probably the deficiency of one or more nutritional growth components. In some antibiotic-producing cultures, the phase of active antibiotic synthesis may be as short as 4-20 hours. However, the production phase may be artificially prolonged by the provision, intermittently or continuously, of a non-inhibitory carbon source. Industrial production of penicillins is thus carried out for up to 200 hours and in some cases for as long as ten days. Some antibiotics, nevertheless, appear to inhibit their own synthesis, and generally the rate of antibiotic production decreases with time and eventually ceases.

Although antibiotic formation usually follows the logarithmic growth phase, this pattern is not universally observed. Nutritional and genetic modifications can transpose the timing of antibiotic synthesis in relation to the phase of vegetative growth. Chloramphenicol [6.1] was the first broad-spectrum antibiotic intro-. duced into medicinal use to inhibit the proliferation of bacteria, e.g. rickettsiae. Present knowledge of chloramphenicol biosynthesis[2] (Scheme 6.1) suggests that the antibiotic may be formed as a result of increased substrate levels of the normal intermediates of aromatic amino-acid biosynthesis, when other pathways requiring these intermediates are partially or wholly closed. Chloramphenicol production is a variable metabolic activity of *Streptomyces venezuelae*; in the defined medium, cultures grow slowly but produce relatively large amounts of the antibiotic (150 mg/l) during the exponential phase. In these circumstances, chloramphenicol [6.1] is a secondary metabolite whose synthesis is not associated with the idiophase. Analogously, the pattern of ergot alkaloid synthesis[3] by *Claviceps paspali* is strongly influenced by the growth rate of the culture.

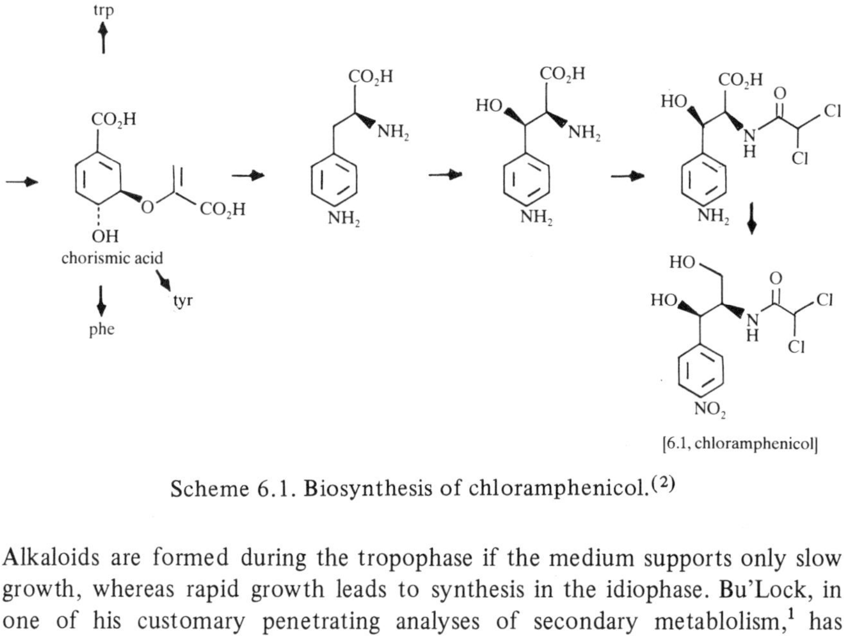

Scheme 6.1. Biosynthesis of chloramphenicol.[2]

Alkaloids are formed during the tropophase if the medium supports only slow growth, whereas rapid growth leads to synthesis in the idiophase. Bu'Lock, in one of his customary penetrating analyses of secondary metablolism,[1] has drawn attention to the thoroughly documented case of the mould *Penicillium urticae* and its synthesis of the mycotoxin patulin (Fig. 6.4). This metabolite is derived from the polyketide 6-methylsalicylic acid by a complex network of reactions which involve a series of key intermediates. However, by manipulating the nutritional state and environmental history of a given *Penicillium urticae* strain, different intermediates of patulin biosynthesis (Fig. 6.4) can be influenced to predominate. The final 'fingerprint' of metabolites which is produced is thus seen to be as much a consequence of phenotypic as genotypic factors. These, and similar, results suggest that any generalized classification of microbial secondary metabolites in relation to the growth phase of the producing organism should perhaps be treated with caution.[1]

Although the picture is less clearly delineated, the same general type of relationship between secondary metabolism, differentiation, and the developmental processes, is believed also to exist in higher plants.[4] Whilst there is no evidence (so far as the author is aware) that habitat changes affect the *qualitative* distribution of plant secondary metabolites, growing conditions can have a marked effect on their *quantitative* distribution.

The plant kingdom still makes an important contribution to the chemical industry as a source of commercially valuable natural products, and the possibility of exploitation of plant tissue cultures as an alternative to whole plants for the production of such secondary metabolites is clearly an attractive proposition. Over the past decade, this area of research has developed to the stage where some twenty cell cultures have been described which produce yields of secondary products similar to those found in the parent plant, e.g. the alkaloids ajmalicine and serpentine from *Catharanthus roseus* and nicotine from *Nicotiana rustica*. In the overall context of secondary metabolism, it is of interest to note some of the features which have emerged from studies of secondary metabolism in plant tissue cultures. During the initial developments with secondary metabolite producing tissue cultures, a particular problem was the apparent need for tissue or organ differentiation as a prerequisite to natural product synthesis. Recent work, however, suggests that natural product synthesis may, under the correct conditions of growth and nutrient supply, be initiated without the need for cell differentiation. The cells in these cultures clearly contain, and are able to transcribe, the information necessary for the production and accumulation of secondary metabolites. Observations such as this support the view of Bu'Lock 'that the potential secondary metabolic activities of an organism are as much a part of its genetic complement as the coding for activities manifest during growth and replication'. The question as to how this potential for secondary metabolite formation is activated remains, as with micro-organisms, uncertain, but it may similarly be linked to nutrient limitations.

Plant tissue-cultures that do not produce secondary metabolites—and at the moment this is probably the greater proportion of tissue-cultures—may possess the genetic information but are unable to use it under the conditions of cell culture.[6] Alternatively, they may simply have lost the capacity for secondary product biosynthesis. For some cell tissue-cultures there is clear evidence that under the conditions of growth only part of the genetic information necessary for secondary metabolite production is expressed. Thus, in cell suspension cultures of *Baptisia australis* only those tetracyclic quinolizidine alkaloids which occur in the biosynthetic sequence (as identified in the whole plant) accumulated in the culture (Scheme 6.2). The principal alkaloid metabolized in tissue culture[7] is lupanine [6.2], and it was therefore concluded that the other alkaloids found in the whole plant, such as tinctorine [6.4] and anagyrine [6.3], are derived sequentially from lupanine [6.2]. Similarly, in *Quercus robur*, leaves of the whole plant metabolize[8] a series of complex

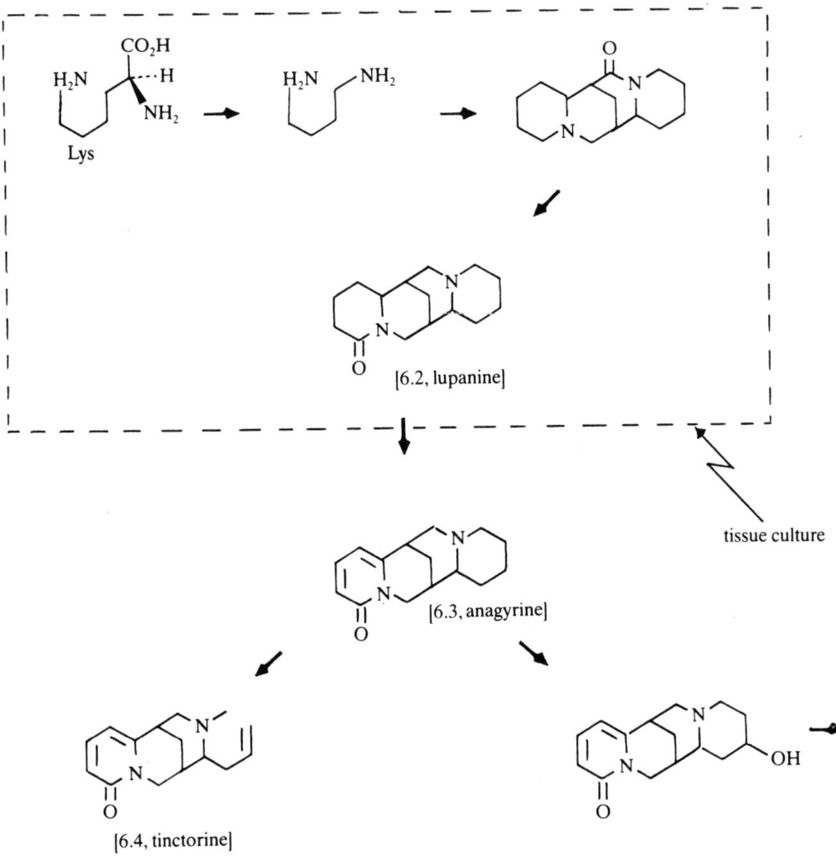

Scheme 6.2. Biosynthesis of quinolizidine alkaloids in *Baptisia*.[7]

hexahydroxydiphenoyl esters [6.6][6.7][6.8] (Scheme 6.3), whose synthesis appears to be based on the initial formation of β-penta-O-galloyl-D-glucose [6.5]. However, in callus tissue culture, *Quercus robur* produces only small quantities of the key ester [6.5], gallic acid, and pyrogallol, and none of the further complex phenolic metabolites furnished by the whole plant ([6.6], [6.7], [6.8], etc.). In kind, these results are similar to those of Bu'Lock with the fungus *Gibberella fujikuroi*. Here the observations were consistent with the view that different pathways of secondary biosynthesis become progressively active at different levels of nutrient depletion[9]; their characteristic products appear in close succession. Thus whilst the expression of secondary metabolism is often growth-linked, it takes place progressively rather than in a simple 'on-off' manner.

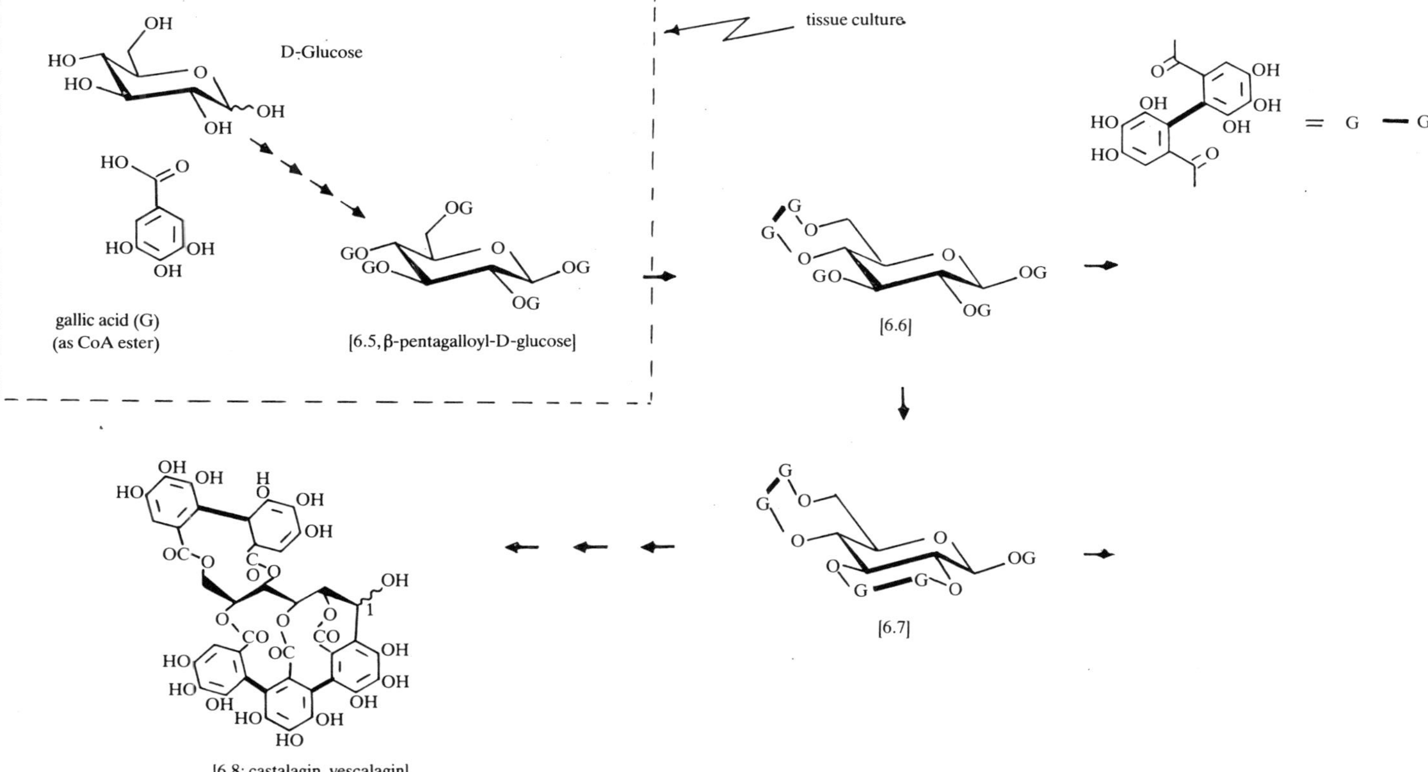

Scheme 6.3. Gallic acid metabolism in *Quercus robur*.[8]

6.2 The role of secondary metabolism—some suggestions

The question of the general role of secondary metabolism in the life of plants and micro-organisms is one to which investigators have addressed themselves with increasing frequency over the past quarter of a century. It is a question which has stimulated continued debate, speculation, mild controversy, and frustation.[5] Many interesting and useful suggestions have been advanced, but the debate has been inconclusive and the question remains essentially unresolved. Several propositions centre on the suggestion that it is the processes of secondary metabolism and not, in the general case, the secondary metabolities themselves which are of importance to the organism. An early idea, advanced by Woodruff[10] and later elaborated and extended by Weinberg in relation to the microbial synthesis of antibiotics, was that these metabolites are normal products of metabolism whose formation is induced by the abnormal stress which results from the limitation to normal growth patterns in the microbial cell. This hypothesis envisages secondary metabolism as an overflow process which results from unbalanced growth, and secondary metabolites as shunt metabolites produced in order to reduce abnormal concentrations of normal cellular constituents. A variation on this theory of unbalanced growth is the suggestion that secondary metabolism is a means of detoxification, where normal intermediates in metabolism reach concentrations toxic to the producing cell. The organism responds by diversion of the intermediate to a less toxic secondary product which may be expelled into the environment or secreted in the cell. Related to these viewpoints, but less clearly defined, is the suggestion that secondary metabolites are merely waste products of metabolism in phylogenetically less advanced organisms. Metabolic inefficiency is, it seems, aesthetically displeasing and explanations such as these have not won the general approval of biologists. This dissatisfaction has led to the search for other ideas. Bu'Lock has developed an intriguing but related proposal of this genre.[5] He has speculated that secondary metabolism serves to maintain basic metabolism in circumstances when its normal substrates, through nutritional imbalances and depletions, cannot be exploited for normal cellular growth and replication. By the formation of enzymes designed to execute the processes of secondary metabolism, the network of enzymes functional in primary metabolism within the organism would continue to operate until such time as circumstances were propitious for renewed metabolic activity and growth.

These suggestions, it should be emphasized, do not exclude the possibility, indeed probability, that the distinctive properties of individual secondary metabolites have, over the course of evolution, secured a particular niche for an organism in the living world. As Brian[11] first noted, the present-day occurrence of antibiotic-producing soil micro-organisms is not incompatible with the view that the capacity to produce mycotoxins is a character conducive to fitness to survive. Similarly, the fact that the tissues of many plants contain unpalatable or toxic metabolites renders them immune to attack by predators—animals, insect, and microbial. Such protection afforded by the metabolites provides, it is assumed, a comparative advantage for the plant and constitutes a secondary benefit. In this sense, these functions which derive from the presence of secondary metabolites are clearly seen as acquired rather than original or predestined.

The physiological response elicited in other organisms are one of the most striking characteristics of many secondary metabolities, and may well provide the clearest indication of the significance of secondary compounds. Although alkaloids are recorded as present in only 10–15 per cent of vascular plants, many distinctive properties of plants derive from the presence of one or more of these nitrogenous bases. Ephedrine ([6.9] *Ephedra* sp.) is thus the basis of an ancient Chinese herbal remedy for ailments of the respiratory tract, and morphine ([6.10] *Papaver somniferum*) is still one of the most efficacious painkillers known to man. Yet again, the three nitrogenous metabolites [6.11] [6.12][6.13] are principally responsible for the familiar sting inflicted by the nettle (*Urtica dioica*). The characteristic astringency of many fruit (archetypally the unripe persimmon), wines, and prepared beverages such as tea, derives from the presence of complex polyphenols in the tissue or extract. Their interaction with the glycoproteins of the mouth produces, it is believed, the astringent sensation. A quite analogous complexation of phenols with proteins forms the basis of the age-old trade of leather manufacture from raw animal skins using infusions of plant materials (e.g. oak mast and bark).

[6.9]

[6.10]

[6.11]

[6.12]

[6.13]

Although such physiological activities may not have been the most significant ones in evolutionary terms, in recent years consideration of these characteristics has led quite logically to attempts to evaluate the selectionary advantage which the presence of such secondary metabolites may confer on plants and micro-organisms. This has been reflected in a growing interest and enthusiasm for both chemical and biochemical facets of ecology. Stahl (1888) appears to have been the first to suggest that some of the chemical substances found in plants may have evolved for protection against attack by herbivores. In his pioneering essay, Stahl concluded that 'the animal world which surrounds the plants deeply influenced not only their morphology but also their chemistry'. The idea lay dormant until Fraenkel[12] (1959) outlined the evidence which indicates that insect host-finding and feeding habits are largely under the influence of various plant secondary metabolites. Others have more recently developed this line of reasoning principally to provide an explanation for the bewildering diversity found today in both flowering plants and insects. Ehrlich and Raven[13] thus concluded that secondary substances play the leading role in determining the patterns of plant utilization. They further suggested a pattern of co-evolution in which plants and insects continually adapt to changes in each other. Janzen[14] has further stated quite explicitly that 'natural selection serves as a mechanism by which a population of herbivores may call forth *de novo* the evolution of a biosynthetic pathway producing compounds toxic to the herbivore'. However, as the evolutionary mechanisms for the acquisition of novel biosynthetic capabilities remain largely unresolved, these ideas have not found universal acceptance.[15] In this context, the view that selective herbivore pressures on several alternative and simultaneously-operational metabolic pathways may well increase the proportion of one of these, appears a more reasonable basis for the exploration of plant–herbivore interactions.

Nevertheless, the general thrust of these ideas has been embraced enthusiastically by many biologists, and particularly by those involved in the rapidly-developing science of ecology. Others have developed and extended the original concepts such that today a general view is emerging in many quarters that the formation of secondary metabolites by plants is as a response to an ecological challenge, and that much of the purpose of their synthesis lies in their development as agents for defence, etc., in the plants' fight for survival. The evidence for this view is, however, often more circumstantial than factual in nature, and a world of caution is appropriate. In this context, the purported role of polyphenols (syn. vegetable tannins) as repellents for a range of predators is frequently and widely cited. The relevant physiological character is considered to be their astringency, based on their ability to complex with proteinaceous materials. This may render plant tissues unpalatable to a predator by precipitating salivary proteins, decrease their nutritional value, or, by immobilizing enzymes, impede the invasion of the host by predators or parasites. However, if the ability of various polyphenols to complex with and precipitate proteins is accurately compared, some surprising results emerge. Thus, in the leaves of species of oak (*Quercus*), the two polyphenols [6.8*a*] and [6.8*b*], end-products of a biosynthetic sequence (Fig. 6.3), overwhelmingly predominate, and presumably the astringent nature of oak-leaf tissue is in large part attributable to these metabolites. However, the ability of these rigid inflexible molecules to complex with proteins is substantially diminished when compared to that of their biosynthetic precusor β-penta-O-galloyl-D-glucose ([6.5] Fig. 6.3). Assuming that the capacity of polyphenols to deter herbivores is measured by their ability to complex with proteins, then in defence terms the synthesis of [6.8*a*] and [6.8*b*] from [6.5] is *per se* counterproductive. This type of evidence suggests that the retention of polyphenolic synthesis by plants may, indeed, confer an advantage and may well be the basis of certain selective pressures—but such protection probably bestows only a secondary benefit on the plant. Polyphenols constitute a group of higher plant natural products of great structural diversity and wide phylogenetic distribution. It is as well to remember that such structural diversity and proliferation may alternatively be viewed, as Bu'Lock has noted in the related context of microbial secondary metabolism[1] . . . 'as a result of there being very little selection pressure on their identity; i.e. the products bring no *great* advantage or disadvantage'.

The 'Janzen' view of secondary metabolism is based on the proposition that plants have evolved an armoury of chemical defences related to the risks which they face.[16] It is appropriate in this connection to make some passing reference to phytoalexins,[17] which are secondary metabolites and defence substances with microbial properties produced by plants. The studies of Muller and Borger on the *Phytophthora* resistance of potatoes led to the first decisive experiments and evidence in this field.[17] One of the essential findings of this work was that the potato plant defended itself against the invading parasite by sacrificing the infected layers of tissues. During this process, a defence substance—a phyto-alexin (*phyton* = plant; *alexin* = to defend)—is synthesized. A range of investigations shows that the ability to synthesize phytoalexins—a form of secondary metabolism—is widespread in the plant kingdom, and may be induced by viruses, by pathogenic and by non-pathogenic micro-organisms. Typical examples of phytoalexins are rishitin [6.14], potatoes—*Solanum tuberosum* infected by *Phytophthora infestans* and medicarpin [6.15], red clover, *Trifolium pratense*. The ability to synthesize phytoalexins seems to be an effective way in which some plants can limit the growth of non-pathogenic micro-organisms. The hypothesis that plants recognize products of microbial origin, and that this then induces phytoalexin synthesis, is an attractive one. Albersheim[18] has recently isolated an elicitor from the mycelial cell walls of *Phytophthora megasperma* var. *sojae* (abbreviated as Pms) which induced the synthesis of the phytoalexin glyceolin [6.16] in various tissues of soyabean. The average molecular weight of the Pms elicitor is 100 000 and it possesses a β-1,3-glucose structure substituted at C-6 with additional sugar residues.

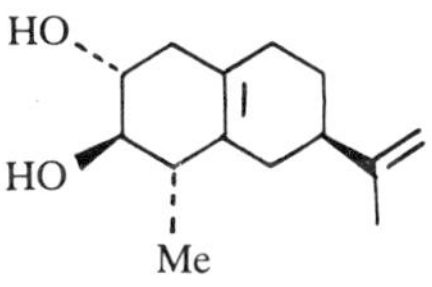

[6.14] 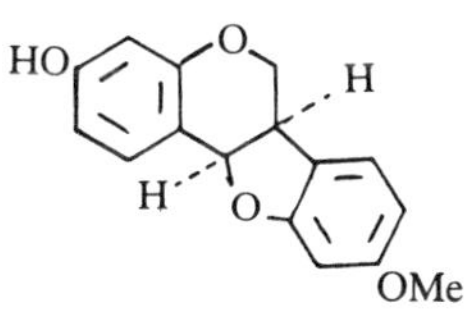   [6.15] 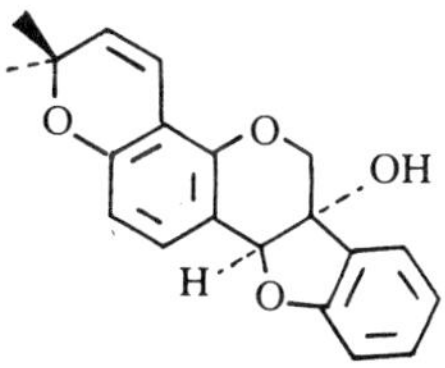   [6.16]

However, there is as yet no generally accepted view of the importance—indeed, perhaps relevance—of phytoalexins in the disease resistance of plants. Exposure of plants to a variety of externally-imposed stresses—cold, ultraviolet light and chemical agents—can also induce phytoalexin synthesis. In every case, the stress produces a profound change in the metabolism of the host plant, and stress metabolites, which are also phytoalexins, are synthesized. This continuing uncertainty as to their true role in plant metabolism is most eloquently signified by the title of a recent authoritative review[17]—'Phytoalexins, chemical defence substances of higher plants?'

6.3 Toxicity and storage of secondary metabolites

Many secondary products thus display either growth-limiting or toxic properties towards foreign organisms, and the problem as to how producer organisms avoid autotoxicity[19] is an intrinsically significant one which has frequently been raised. Woodruff first posed the question,[10] in a microbiolgical context, when he questioned how antibiotic-producing organisms withstand the action of their own metabolites. In large-scale microbiological practice this may be an important constraint, if the antibiotic-producing culture cannot grow satisfactorily in the presence of its own secondary metabolites. These growth-inhibitory effects are well illustrated with various *Streptomyces* species.[19] Thus, the capacity for fresh growth of certain streptomycin [6.17] producing strains of *Streptomyces griseus* may be reduced by up to 50 per cent with concentrations of the antibiotic as small as 75μg/ml although the normal production levels are of the order of 200 μg/ml. *Streptomyces antibioticus* strains capable of producing as much as 120 μg/ml of actinomycin [6.18] suffer 50 per cent inhibition of fresh growth from an inoculation when actinomycin levels are only 4 μg/ml. Similar effects have been noted with *Streptomyces niveus* and the antibiotic novobiocin [6.19]. Other antibiotics which inhibit growth of their respective producing organisms are oxytetracycline [6.20] and chlortetracycline [6.21], chloramphenicol [6.1], neomycin, and polymyxin. Mutation to enhance the resistance of the organism to the mycotoxin and to improve yields is the normal approach to overcome or limit this problem on the industrial scale of antibiotic production. Where the antibiotic has no unique relationship to the producing organism then the latter is resistant to its effects. *Penicillium chrysogenum* thus lacks the normal target—the bacterial cell wall—for pencillin action ([6.22a] penicillin N). The antibiotic-producing cultures of this organism are thus inert to the microbial activity of this particular secondary metabolite.

In discussions of this nature it is timely to recall the words of Sergei Winogradsky (1928), who emphasized that the activities of soil bacteria in the laboratory are no criterion for their behaviour in the soil complex. Mutation is the chief factor responsible for the hundred- to thousand-fold increases which have been obtained in the production of antibiotics from the point of their initial

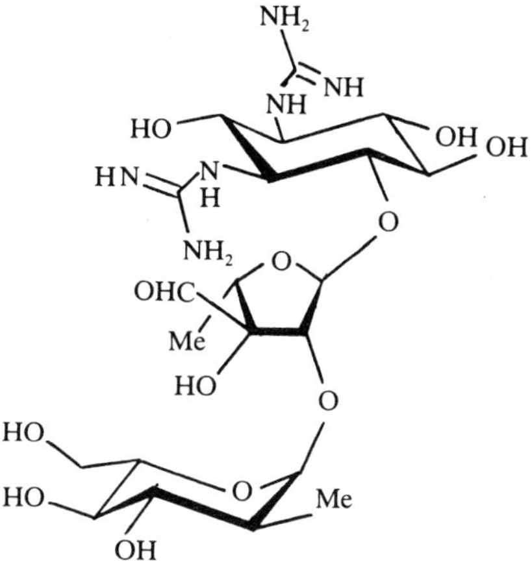

[6.17]

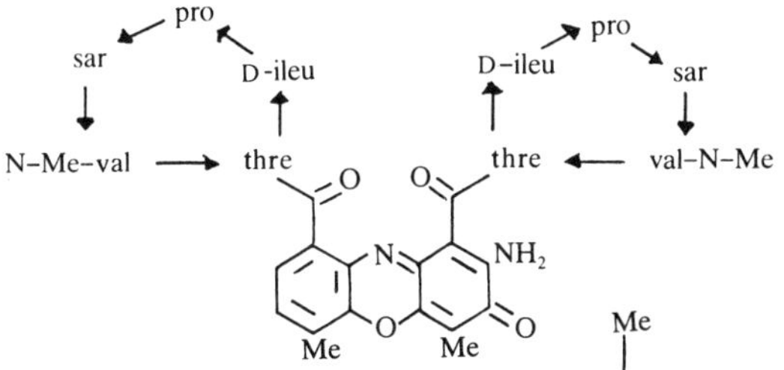

sar ← pro ← D-ileu   D-ileu → pro → sar

N–Me–val ⟶ thre   thre ← val–N–Me

[6.18]

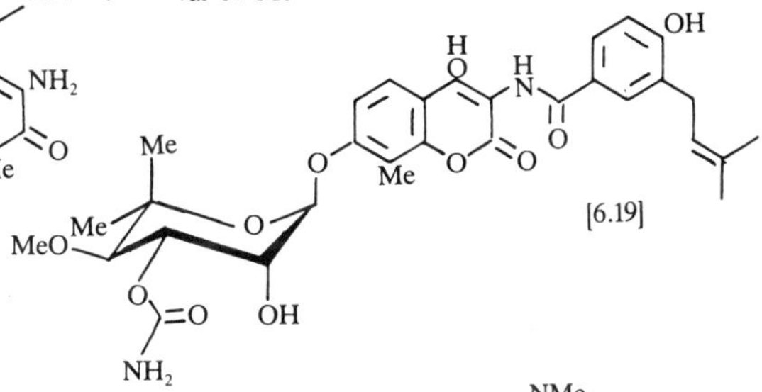

[6.19]

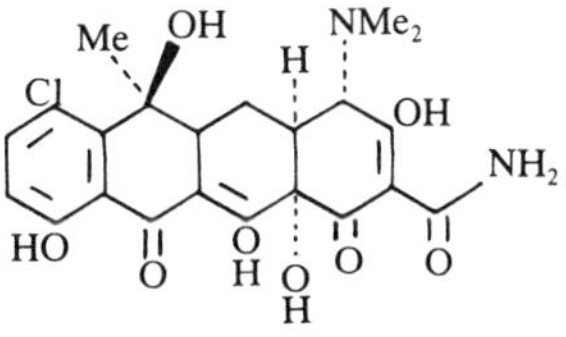

[6.20]

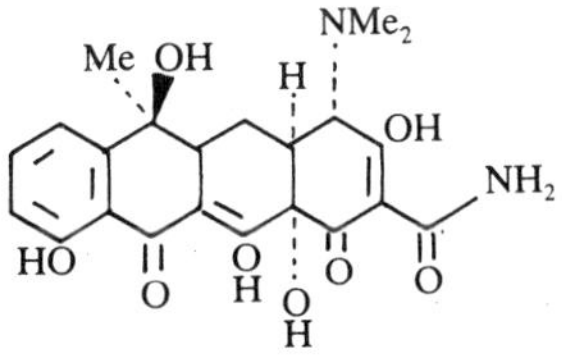

[6.21]

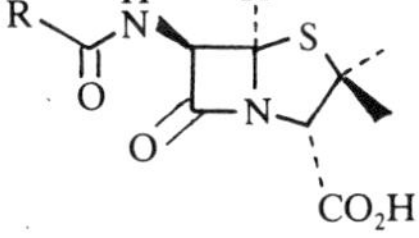

[6.22a] R =

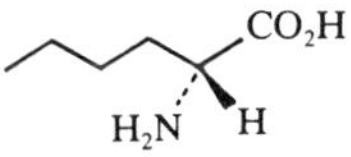

[6.22b] R =

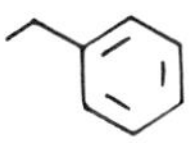

discovery in micro-organisms.[20] In the case of penicillin G [6.22*b*], levels of the antibiotic produced in the culture fluid of mutants of the Wisconsin strain of *Penicillium chrysogenum* Q–176 were, for example, raised from $\sim$5 mg/l in 1949 to $\sim$10 000 mg/l in 1970. Such laboratory cultures perfectly fit Winogradsky's eloquent description of 'domestic hot-house organisms'. They are perhaps not the best vehicles for studies designed to determine the function, from the micro-organism point of view, of antibiotics.

There is, nevertheless, ample evidence in the plant kingdom that many secondary metabolites are significant factors in the plant's interactions with its own natural habitat.[21] In many cases, secondary products perturb the growth of other plants in the same locality. Normally, the effect is a deleterious one, but the phenomenon is generally referred to as allelopathy. A ubiquitous shrub of the chaparral is *Andenostoma fasciculatum* (Rosaceae). Under the mature shrub, few herbaceous species can grow, and Muller and his collaborators have presented[21] strong evidence to suggest that toxic materials, leached by rainfall from the leaves, are responsible—at least in part—for poor herb growth in the vicinity of the shrub. The leachate of *Andenostoma* foliage yielded many readily identifiable and familiar plant secondary phenolic metabolites, p-coumaric acid [6.23], ferulic acid [6.24], p-hydroxybenzoic acid [6.25], and arbutin (hydroquinone-β-D-glucoside [6.26]). In bioassays, all these substances showed toxicity to seedling growth and inhibited germination. Similar reports of the toxicity of coumarin [6.27] and its derivatives to plant growth have been numerous. Recently, Brown summarized the recorded information.[22] Some stimulatory and inductive changes were noted, but the majority of classified effects refer to inhibitory, repressive, and retarding actions—e.g. germination and tissue growth. Analogously, the presence of volatilized cineole [6.28] and camphor [6.29] in the atmosphere surrounding foliar branches of *Salvia leucophylla* has been established by gas chromatography. The striking toxic effects of these and other simple terpenes on plants has been amply demonstrated. Allelopathy is fundamentally an ecological phenomenon, and in a study of this problem Newman[23] observed that 'there is not often specific selection for allelopathic activity or tolerance of allelopathy, but that these plant properties are better viewed as the fortuitous outcome of characteristics of the plant whose primary reason for existence is not allelopathy'. He concluded that the character should not be viewed in isolation from the other implications of plant secondary metabolism.

Against this background it is perhaps useful to briefly consider how plants themselves avoid suicide.[19] Inherently toxic products synthesized by plants do not appear to inhibit growth or otherwise interfere with the metabolism of the parent plant. In many instances this end-result appears to be achieved by physical removal of the toxic metabolite(s) from the cellular synthetic machinery. This may occur by aerial discharge, as in the case of the volatile monoterpenes of *Salvia leucophylla* (*vide supra*), by precipitation of insoluble salts (e.g. calcium oxalate), or most commonly by physical isolation in the plant cell vacuole. In

[6.23, R = H]
[6.24, R = OMe]

[6.25]

[6.26]

[6.27]

[6.28]

[6.29]

many mature plants, the vacuole is thought to be the sub-cellular site to which most secondary metabolites are translocated and stored. Direct evidence which confirms this view comes from histochemical staining and from the application of techniques which allow the isolation of individual plant cell organelles. In the case of dark-grown Sorghum shoots, it has been shown that at least 95 per cent of the cyanogenic glucoside dhurrin [6.30] in the shoots is present in the vacuole.

[6.30, dhurrin]

6.4 Secondary metabolism—chemical characteristics

The use of isotopic tracers to delineate pathways of secondary metabolism has been attended with remarkable success over the past twenty-five years. Nevertheless, in this context, the logic of working with enzymes to define metabolic pathways and to determine patterns of control has been repeatedly stressed. Our present knowledge and appreciation of this aspect of secondary metabolism remains very much at the cinderella stage. Much of the machinery of secondary metabolism in plants and micro-organisms has proved to be surprisingly inaccessible using conventional biochemical techniques, although there have been some recent notable successes—with polyketides, flavonoids and some alkaloids—which are described below. Prior to such a discussion, it is pertinent to briefly recall one outstanding and quite general characteristic— namely, the biosynthetic prodigality associated with secondary metabolism; the diversity of structures all derived by elegant perambulations and blind alleys from one major chemical theme. This facet above all best illustrates the general nature of secondary metabolism. Any explanation of this phenomenon must therefore seek to rationalize such apparent extravagance and to show why it is both possible and permissible. The remaining discussion both here and in the following chapter concentrates on this particular general aspect of secondary metabolism, and at appropriate points discreetly advances some tentative proposals!

6.5 Secondary metabolism—enzymology

A general characteristic of secondary metabolism, to which at this stage inevitably only circumstantial evidence points, is the relatively low specificity of many enzymes involved in secondary biosynthetic pathways, or alternatively the existence of a large number of isoenzymes with closely related structural and stereochemical specificities. We are accustomed to think in terms of the extraordinary specificity of enzymes, since our views are generally conditioned by our knowledge of the key enzymes of primary metabolism, and the long-standing concept of the biochemical unity of all forms of life. Jensen[24] has pointed out, however, that primitive enzymes probably possessed a very broad specificity which permitted them to react with a range of related substrates, enabling the ancestral cell to function with limited enzyme resources. This view was developed in part from a consideration of different biosynthetic pathways which exist for certain α-amino-acids.

Enzymes of secondary metabolism appear to possess something of this character. In many cases this means that not all the metabolic traffic along a given pathway is proceeding by the same route from starting material to end-product. Different chemical operations may be carried out in various sequences, so that the system resembles a metabolic grid rather than a linear pathway. Bu'Lock has been largely responsible for the development of this idea in relation to aromatic polyketide biosynthesis in *Penicillium urticae*. A number of micro-fungi can be grown so as to produce 6-methylsalicylic acid [6.33] and a standard strain of *Penicillium urticae* can be manipulated to give [6.33], *m*-cresol [6.34], gentisyl alcohol [6.35], or the mycotoxin patulin [6.36] as the predominant metabolite. The ways in which these and other polyketide metabolites are interrelated in the form of a metabolic grid is shown in Scheme 6.4.

This apparently decreased sensitivity of the enzymes of secondary metabolism to variations in the substitution pattern of substrate molecules is also illustrated in a number of other examples. In studies of the biosynthesis of the tetracycline class of antibiotics, mutants of *Streptomyces aurocofaciens* and *Streptomyces rimosus* were obtained which had lost their ability to synthesize any substantial quantity of tetraycline antibiotics.[26] Deductions concerning the biosynthetic pathway to the tetracyclines were made from the nature of the

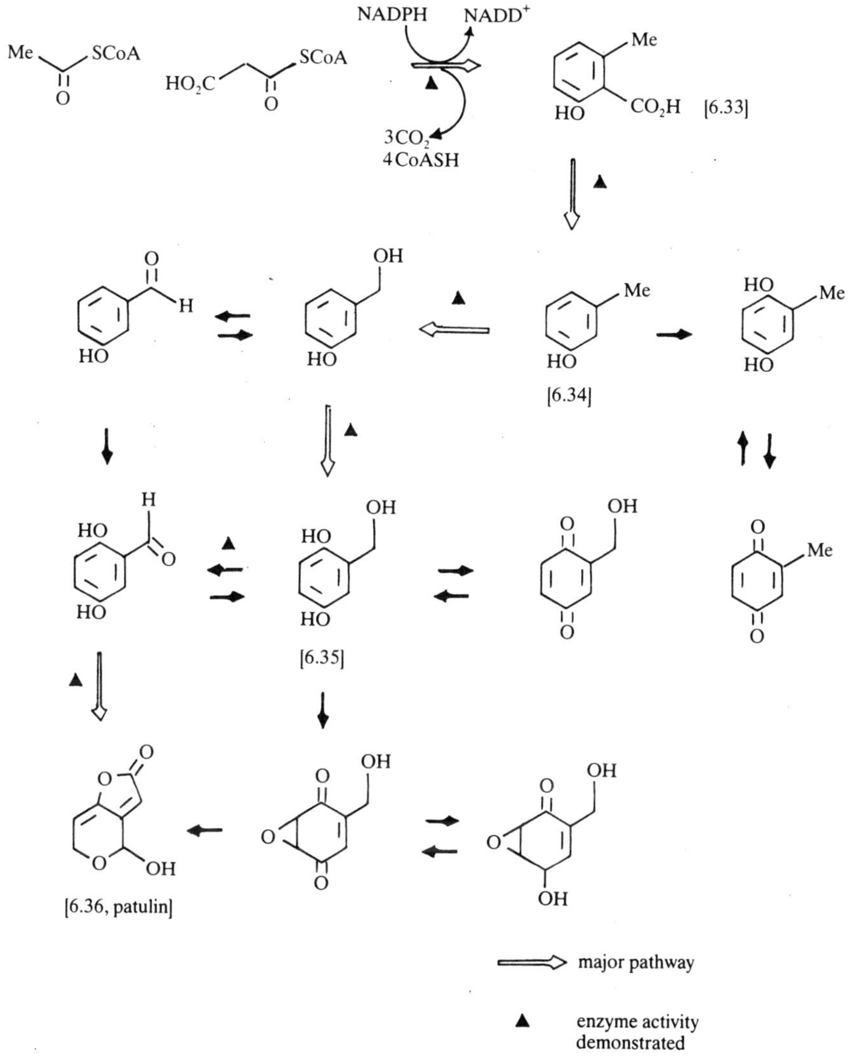

Scheme 6.4. Aromatic polyketide biosynthesis in *Pencillin urticae*. Relationships between metabolites and the biosynthetic pathway to patulin [6.36].[25]

mutant metabolites and from the pattern of co-synthesis between pairs of blocked mutants. With the latter technique, substantial amounts of one or more tetracyclines were formed in the mixed fermentation even when each mutant grown in isolation gave no appreciable quantity of tetracyclines. It was assumed that in the co-synthesis either the intermediates from the mutant with the later block in the biosynthetic pathway were transferred to the mutant with the earlier block, or, alternatively, that the missing facility from either mutant was transferred to the other, such that the co-operative biosynthesis of the normal product of the parent strain could take place. In this way, the major route of chlotetracycline [6.39] biosynthesis was deduced (Scheme 6.5). Many of these deductions were, however, complicated by the relatively broad specificity of the enzymes involved in tetracycline biosynthesis. Thus, mutants blocked in chlorination produce tetracycline, the non-chlorinated analogue of [6.39], and hence chlorination (step '*b*') is not obligatory for subsequent amination, N-methylation, C-6 hydroxylation and reduction (steps '*c*'–'*f*'). Similarly, mutants lacking the C-6 methylase (step '*a*') produce 6-demethyltetracyclines rather than accumulate the intermediate [6.38], and mutants unable to form sufficient quantities of malonamyl CoA [6.37]—a starting material for tetracycline biosynthesis— produce tetracyclines with a 2-acetyl rather than a 2-carboxamide substituent. Thus, in these mutant *Streptomyces* species, the absence of a pathway enzyme does not lead (as in a primary metabolic pathway) to simple accumulation of an intermediate. Enzymes, which in principle function later in the sequence, still operate with the production of a shunt metabolite.

Investigation of the mechanism of generation of the penicillin ring system has been considerably facilitated by the isolation of a cyclase enzyme in a cell-free extract of *Cephalosporium acremonium*. The enzyme—isopenicillin N synthetase—has a molecular weight of 37 000 and is active in the presence of ferrous sulphate, dithiothreitol, ascorbic acid, catalase and oxygen. It efficiently converts the tripeptide (ACV, L-α-aminoadipyl-L-cysteinyl-D-valine [6.40]) to iso-penicillin N. The cyclase enzyme has, however, been shown additionally to be capable of accepting and transferring structurally-modified substrates into new penicillins.[27] Thus, the modified tripeptide substrates [6.41] [6.42] were converted to the corresponding penam derivatives [6.44] [6.45]. Although the extent of conversion observed was much less than the virtually quantitative yield from the natural substrate (ACV [6.40]) the results illustrate the relatively broad structural specificity of the key cyclase enzyme. Rather surprisingly, when the pseudo-substrate ([6.42] L-α-aminoadipyl-L-cysteinyl-D-α-aminobutyrate) was incubated with the enzyme the cepham [6.43] was isolated. The ratio of penam to cepham was $\sim$3:1. It was concluded, therefore, that the enzyme isopenicillin-*N*-synthetase, in addition to being able to accept structurally-modified tripeptide substrates, is also able to effect both five- and six-membered oxidative cyclizations with such precursors. The balance between these alternative pathways may well be influenced by the enhanced conformational mobility of the terminal *n*-butyric acid residue in the enzyme-substrate complex.

Finally, in this context, attention should be drawn to the two hundred or more non-protein amino-acids which are synthesized by higher plants as part of their rich diversity of secondary metabolites.[28] Many of these non-protein amino-acids are related structurally to the amino-acids which are integral parts of common proteins. Excellent examples are L-canavanine (Scheme 6.8) [6.52], the guanidinoxy analogue of L-arginine, and *m*-carboxy-L-phenylalanine [6.50]

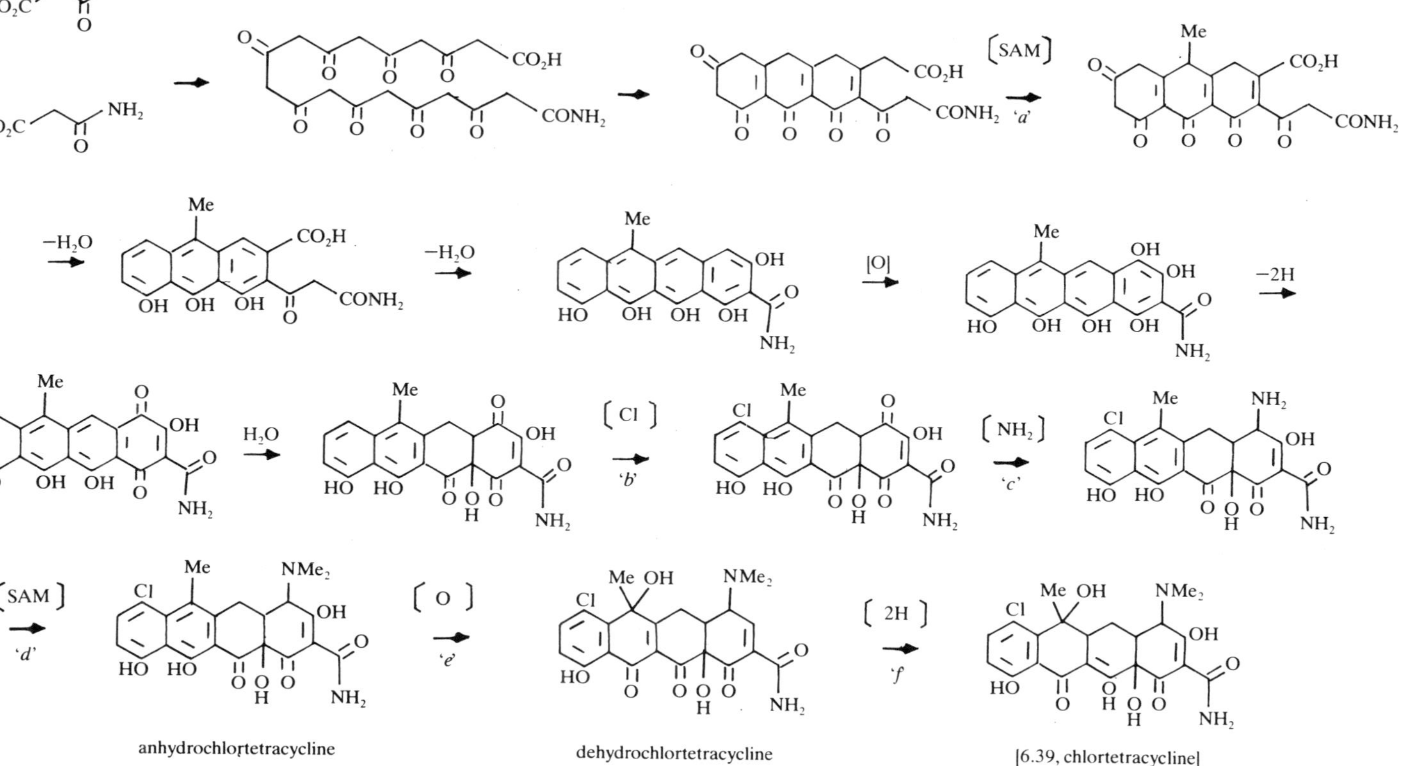

Scheme 6.5. Principal pathway of biosynthesis of chlortetracycline [6.39].

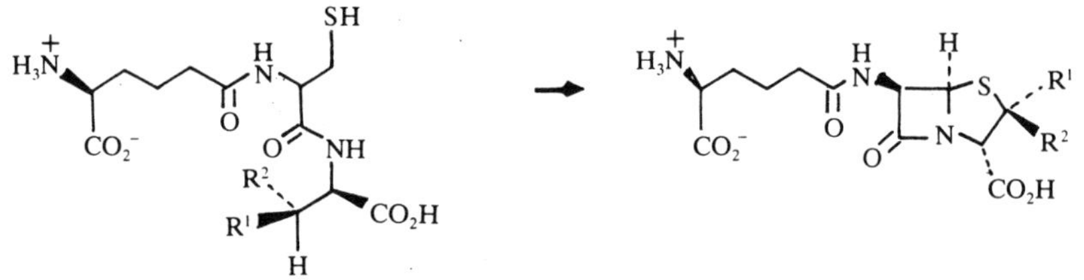

[6.40; R^1 = R^2 = Me]
[6.41; R^1 = Me, R^2 = Et]
[6.42; R^1 = H, R^2 = Me]

[6.43; R^1 = R^2 = Me]
[6.44; R^1 = R^2 = Et]
[6.45; R^1 = H, R^2 = Me]

(i) isopenicillin N synthetase

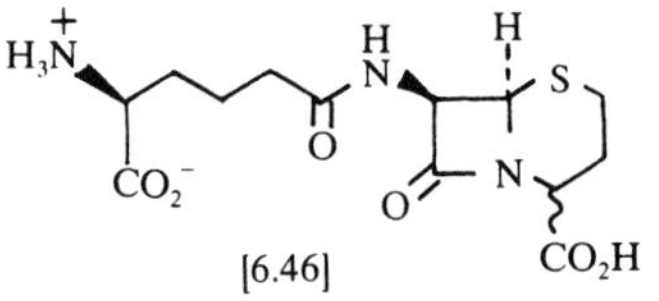

[6.46]

Scheme 6.6. Enzymic transformation related to penicillin biosynthesis.[27]

and *m*-carboxy-L-tyrosine [6.51] analogues respectively of the aromatic amino-acids L-phenylalanine [6.48] and L-tyrosine [6.49]. Fowden[29] has suggested that the metabolic pathways culminating in the synthesis of certain non-protein amino-acids may reflect subtle alteration of the genome responsible for direct-ing the formation of the corresponding protein amino-acids. Larsen[30] has illustrated[29] this idea in the pathways of biosynthesis of the *m*-carboxy aro-matic amino-acids [6.50] and [6.51] as deduced from tracer studies. Thus, L-phenylalanine [6.48] and L-tyrosine [6.49] are derived from chorismic acid [6.46] (Scheme 6.7) whilst their *m*-carboxy counterparts are thought to be synthesized in a corresponding manner from the isomeric substrate, isochorismic acid [6.47] (Scheme 6.7).

Most plants similarly possess the urea-ornithine cycle enzymes as a means of providing for the biosynthesis of L-arginine (Scheme 6.8). Rosenthal[31] has suggested that an entirely analogous pathway—the urea–canaline cycle (Scheme 6.9)—may have its origins as a route of biosynthesis for L-canavanine [6.52] by evolutionary modification of the pre-existing means of production of the amino-acid L-arginine. Rosenthal has established that the urea-ornithine-arginine cycle enzymes are able to sequentially-metabolize the urea–canaline–canavanine intermediates, although it should be borne in mind that these results do not prove that this series of reactions is the sole or even the principal means of L-canavanine [6.52] synthesis *in vivo*.

Further confirmation of this view, that the types of enzymic processes concerned in the biosynthesis of non-protein amino-acids are apparently often

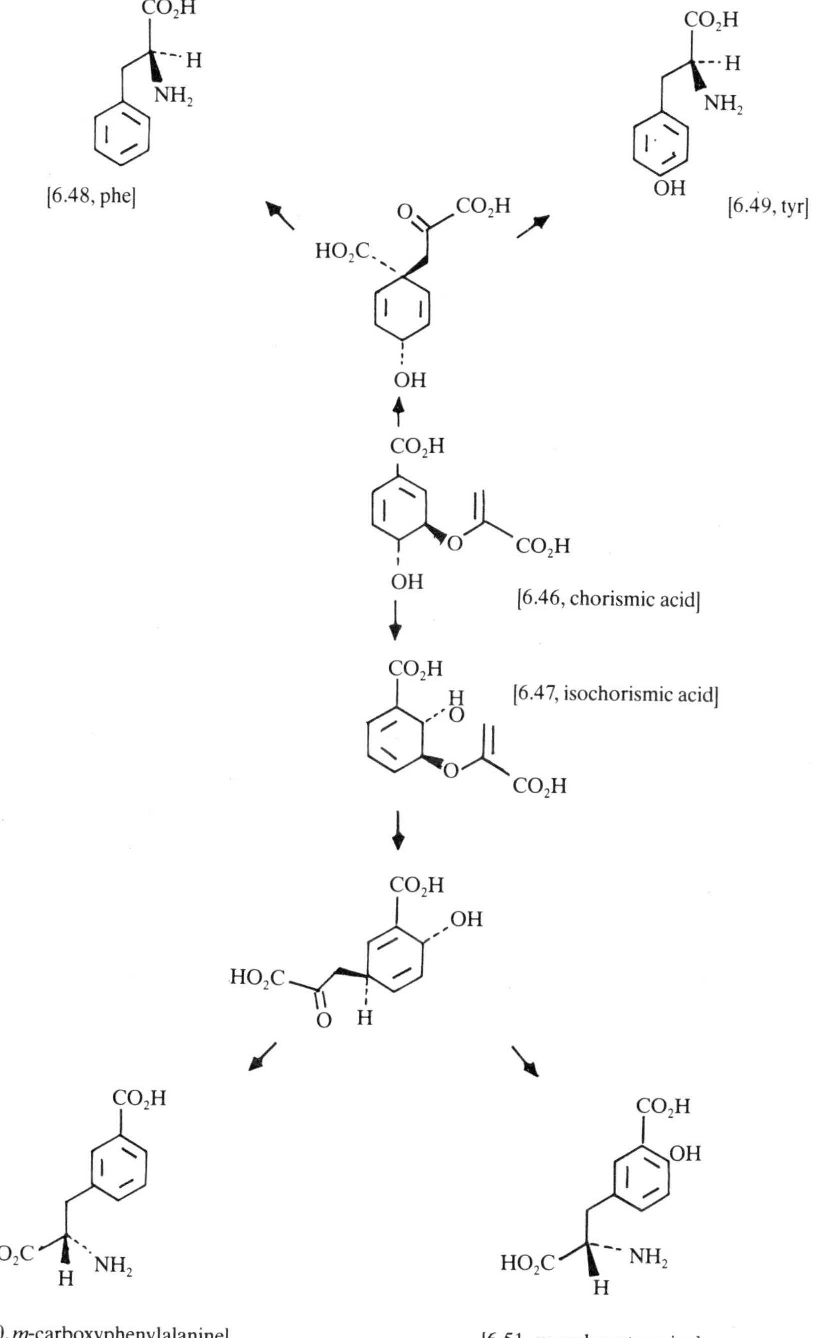

Scheme 6.7. Biosynthesis of aromatic amino-acids in higher plants.[30]

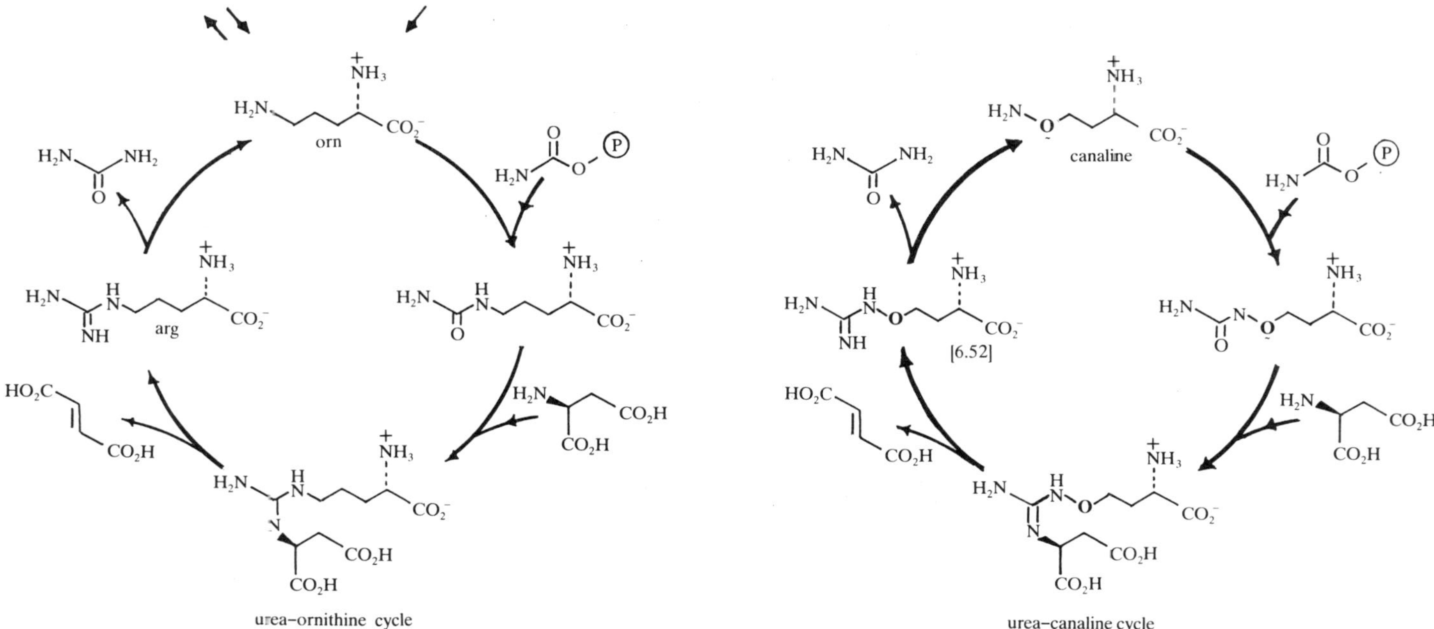

Scheme 6.8. Biosynthesis of canavanine [6.52] in legumes (Rosenthal[31]).

minor deviations from the biosynthesis of related protein amino-acids, is also derived from observations with O-acetyl-L-serine [6.53]. L-Cysteine [6.54] is derived from [6.53] in bacteria, and recent work indicates that the same pathway is utilized for the production of [6.54] in plants. Pathways also lead from O-acetyl-L-serine [6.53] to many of the related but distinctive non-protein α-amino-acids, shown in Scheme 6.9, which are found in plants. The intermediate [6.53] presumably represents a branch-point in higher plant metabolism. Displacement of the acetoxy group in the conventional (biochemical) sense by sulphur leads to L-cysteine. Alternatively, displacement by either carbon or nitrogen nucleophiles gives rise to the various non-protein α-amino-acids.[28, 30]

Although cell-free extracts containing mixtures of enzymes have been prepared in a number of cases, individual enzymes of secondary metabolic pathways have not been widely described. Dimethylallyl-L-tryptophan synthetase—the first enzyme in the biosynthetic pathway to lysergic acid—has been obtained and purified to homogeneity[32] (Scheme 6.10). The enzyme is inhibited by alkaloid end-products agroclavine and elymoclavine, suggesting the possibility of some form of feedback inhibition in the biosynthesis. In *Penicillium patulum*, the enzymology of patulin synthesis (Scheme 6.5) has been studied in detail and several enzymes have been isolated and authenticated.[33] The initial enzyme in the biosynthetic sequence 6-methylsalicylic acid synthetase has been purified to varying degrees, and both Lynen and Scott[34] have proposed a model for the enzyme based upon its many similarities to the fatty acid synthetase. Thus, two sulphydryl groups are envisaged as integral parts of the enzyme complex—one at the periphery and one at the centre. All the reactions are envisaged as occurring on the multi-enzyme complex, with the peripheral sulphydryl group as part of a flexible arm (4'-phospho-pantotheine residue), which brings the group in close juxtaposition to the active site of the enzyme and the growing polyketide chain.

Undifferentiated cell tissue cultures from higher plants have proved to be valuable sources of a number of enzymes, and enzyme activities associated with secondary metabolism. The initial stages of biosynthesis of the terpenoid indole skeleton—one of the most widely encountered in plant alkaloids—has been substantially clarified using enzyme preparations from *Catharanthus roseus* cell suspension cultures.[35] In contrast to previous conclusions, based upon isotopic tracer studies with whole plants, the precursor of monoterpenoid *Catharanthus* alkaloids which arises from the enzymatic condensation of tryptamine [6.55] and secologanin [6.56] is $3\alpha(S)$-strictosidine (isovincoside [6.57]) and not its $3\beta(R)$-epimer (vincoside). Strictosidine [6.57] accumulates in the enzymic synthesis in presence of δ-D-gluconolactone, a β-glucosidase inhibitor, which blocks the cell-free synthesis of ajmalicine [6.59] and its isomers. In the absence of the β-glucosidase inhibitor but in presence of reduce pyridine nucleotide (NADH or NADPH) the biosynthesis proceeds normally through cathenamine [6.58] to ajmalicine [6.59] (Scheme 6.11).

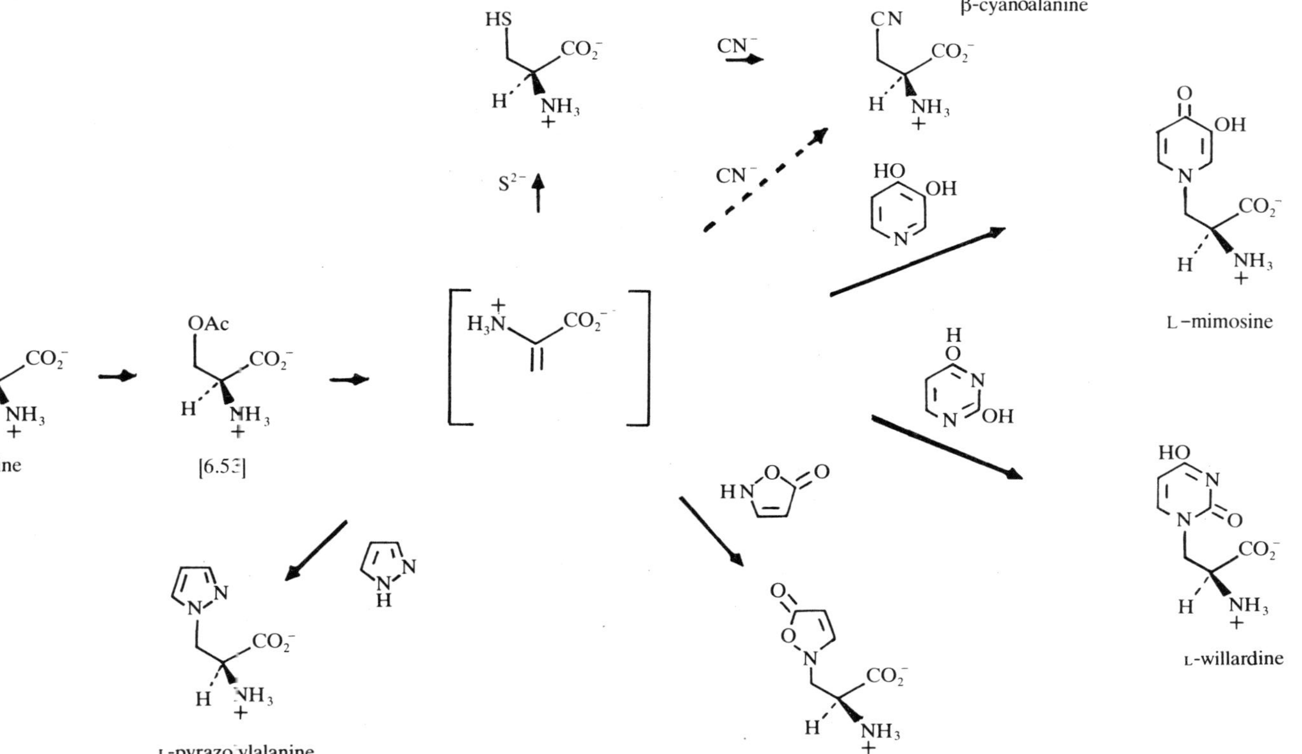

Scheme 6.9. Metabolism of O-acetyl-L-serine [6.53]: biosynthesis of some non-protein α-amino-acids in higher plants.[28, 30]

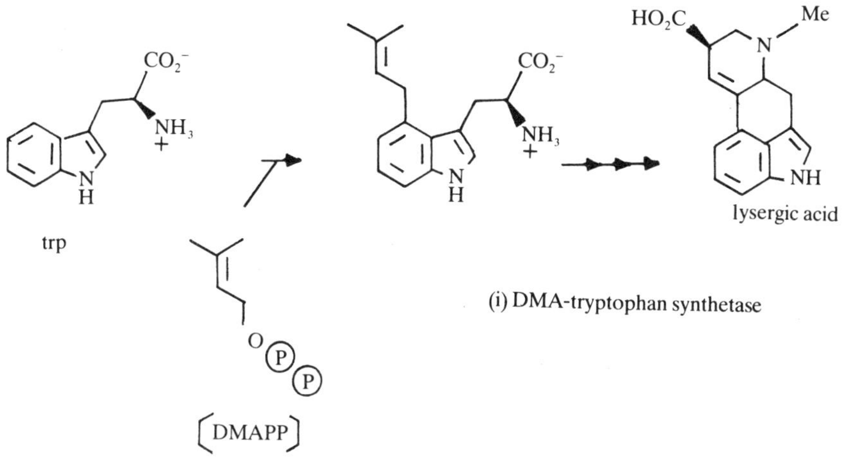

trp

[DMAPP]

(i) DMA-tryptophan synthetase

lysergic acid

Scheme 6.10. Biosynthesis of lysergic acid.[32]

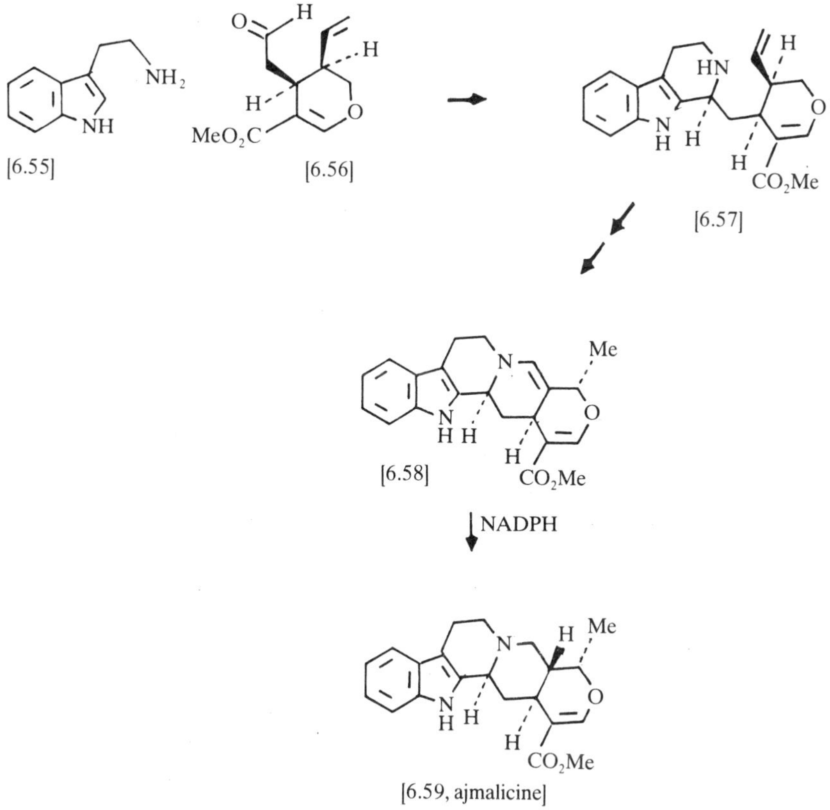

[6.55]

[6.56]

[6.57]

[6.58]

NADPH

[6.59, ajmalicine]

Scheme 6.11. Cell-free biosynthesis of ajmalicine and related indole alkaloids.

One of the most detailed studies of the enzymology of secondary metabolism has been carried out[36] with cell suspension cultures of *Petroselinum hortense* (parsley). Irradiation of the cultures with u.v. light coordinately induces the enzymes of flavonoid metabolism and leads to the rapid production of flavone and flavonol glycosides, principally of apiin [6.60] and graveobioside B (3'-methoxyapiin). The ubiquitous C_{15} flavonoid skeleton is assembled from cinnamate (C_6-C_3) and acetate/malonate ($3 \times C_2$) units, and the enzymes which lead to its formation may be divided into two groups. The first group comprises those concerned with general phenylpropanoid metabolism in higher plants—phenylalanine ammonia lyase (PAL), cinnamate-4-hydroxylase, and p-coumaroyl CoA ligase. The second group of a dozen or more enzymes includes the key chalcone synthase which catalyses the key step in flavonoid biosynthesis—the sequential condensation of three molecules of malonyl CoA with p-coumaroyl CoA (Scheme 6.12).

[6.60]

In cell suspension cultures of parsley, the two groups of enzymes can be clearly distinguished. Rapid increases and subsequent decreases in activity of the group 1 enzymes occur in a strictly coordinated manner when a cell culture is diluted into fresh medium. Both groups of enzymes are sensitive to light and are induced simultaneously when cultures are irradiated. Group 1 enzymes reach maximal activity several hours earlier and decline much more rapidly than enzymes of the second group. The first two enzymes of group 1 display many similarities to the same enzymes of general phenylpropanoid metabolism from other plants. The third enzyme of this sequence, p-coumaroyl CoA ligase, has a marked specificity for *trans*-p-hydroxy-cinnamate as substrate. Its marked regulatory characteristics indicate that this enzyme probably represents a sensitive point of control for the distribution of cinnamoyl CoA esters between different pathways of phenylpropanoid metabolism in plants. The enzyme from parsley is strongly inhibited by AMP and exhibits sigmoidal kinetics for the two co-substrates of p-coumaric acid—ATP and coenzyme A. This behaviour was interestingly (*vide infra*) interpreted in terms of the possible regulation of enzyme activity through the ATP/AMP ratio.

Chalcone synthase catalyses the reaction which is the point of departure of flavonoid biosynthesis from general phenylpropanoid metabolism. The mechanism of sequential addition of three molecules of malonyl CoA with p-coumaroyl CoA is supported by a number of pieces of evidence and is similar to that proposed for fatty acid and polyketide biosynthesis. Thus, under certain *in vitro* assay conditions, products containing one (styryl pyrone) or two (dihydropyrone) acetate/malonate units less than naringenin [6.62] were observed. However rigorously purified, chalcone synthase does not contain an acyl carrier protein nor a pantotheinyl residue directly bound to the enzyme, and it utilizes coenzyme A esters directly as intermediate substrates. Finally, chalcone isomerase converts the chalcone [6.61] to the flavanone, naringenin [6.62]. The enzyme from parsley is quite specific for this pair of substrates and it is noteworthy that in other plants the comparable enzyme often occurs in multiple forms which are probably true isoenzymes with slightly different substrate specificities.

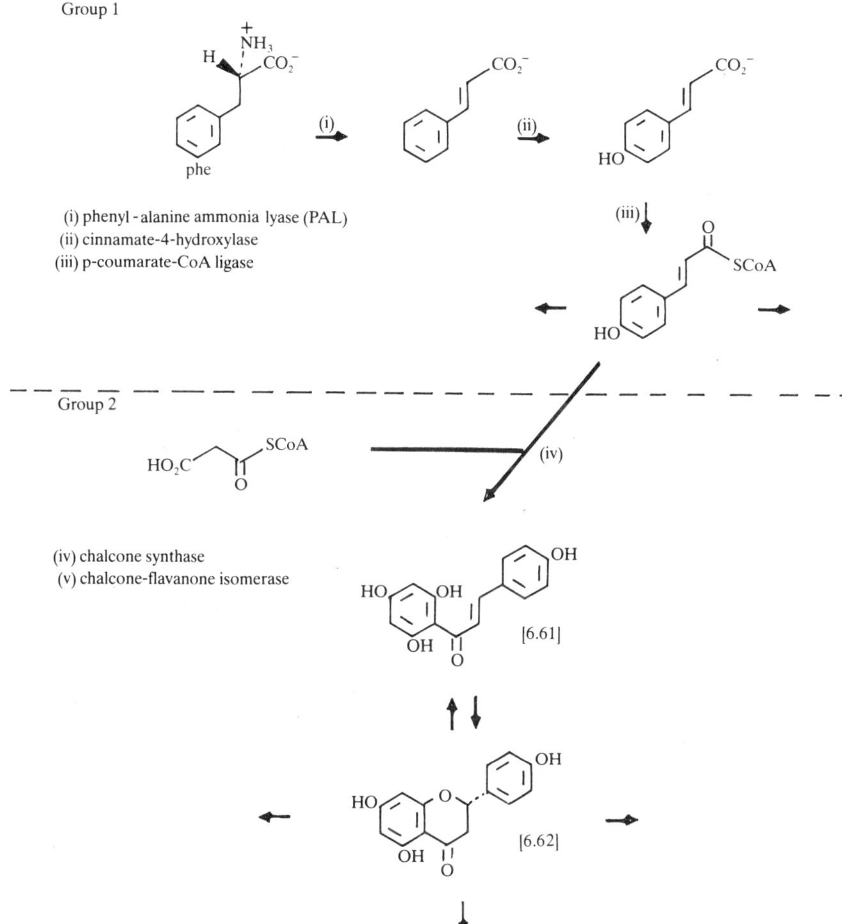

Scheme 6.12. General pathway of flavanoid biosynthesis—*Petroselinum hortense* (parsley).[36]

The work of Hahlbrock and his collaborators[36] with parsley cell cultures points to the way in which enzyme studies in this field should develop, and lead the way ultimately to a better understanding of the factors which regulate and control secondary metabolism in different organisms.

6.6 Regulation of secondary metabolism

Some facets of the methods whereby regulation of secondary metabolism is achieved at the molecular level in some organisms has begun to emerge from these and other studies. In the past few years it has become evident that several microbial antibiotics inhibit their own synthesis (*vide supra*). Examples include chloramphenicol[2] [6.1] where there is feedback repression of the arylamine synthetase—the first enzyme of the biosynthetic branch leading to chloramphenicol—that converts chorismic acid to p-aminophenylalanine[37] (Scheme 6.1). Feedback inhibition and regulation may also occur by way of primary metabolites. Some pathways of antibiotic biosynthesis share the initial part of the pathway of biosynthesis with that of a primary metabolite. In such divergent pathways, the primary metabolite controls, by feedback regulation, enzymes of its own synthesis. If these fall on the common pathway their inhibition may reduce thereby the synthesis of the antibiotic. Thus, lysine and valine both regulate, by this means, penicillin production in *Penicillium chrysogenum*[38] (Scheme 6.13). It is interesting to note that the acetohydroxy acid synthetase of a mutant strain producing large quantities of penicillin was much less sensitive to valine than the same enzyme from a low-producer strain. This suggests a loss of regulatory mechanisms during the industrial selection of high-producer strains.

Analogous observations have been made in the study of the biosynthesis of the polyene macrolide antibiotic candicidin [6.64]. 4-Aminobenzoic acid [6.63] has been identified as the immediate precursor of the aromatic nucleus of candicidin in *Streptomyces griseus*. The branching point of the pathway of aromatic amino-acid biosynthesis—the shikimate pathway—which gives rise to the p-aminobenzoyl unit appears to be chorismic acid [6.64]. Biochemical evidence supports a two-step pathway to 4-aminobenzoic acid from chorismic acid [6.46], although no intermediates have yet been isolated. The biosynthesis of candicidin is inhibited (50 per cent) by a 5 mM mixture of L-tryptophan [6.65], L-tyrosine, and L-phenylalanine, and later work showed the inhibition to be due exclusively to L-tryptophan. It has been suggested[25] that this control is effected by regulation of the 4-aminobenzoic acid synthase of *Streptomyces griseus* by L-tryptophan. This conclusion is based on the well-known inhibition of anthranilic acid synthetase by L-tryptophan, and the fact that, in several organisms, 4-aminobenzoic acid synthase and anthranilic acid synthetase possess several identical sub-units (Scheme 6.14).

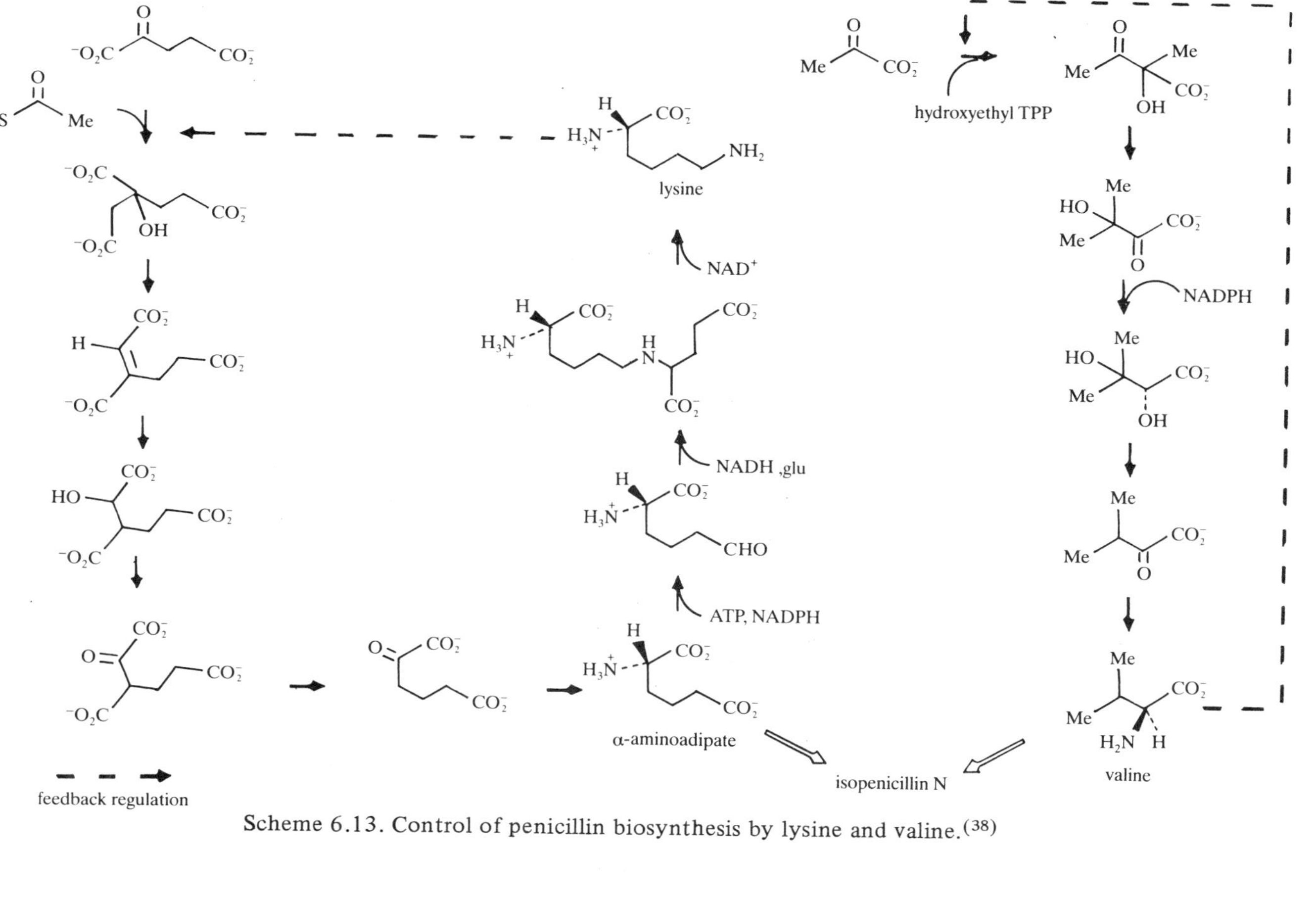

Scheme 6.13. Control of penicillin biosynthesis by lysine and valine.(38)

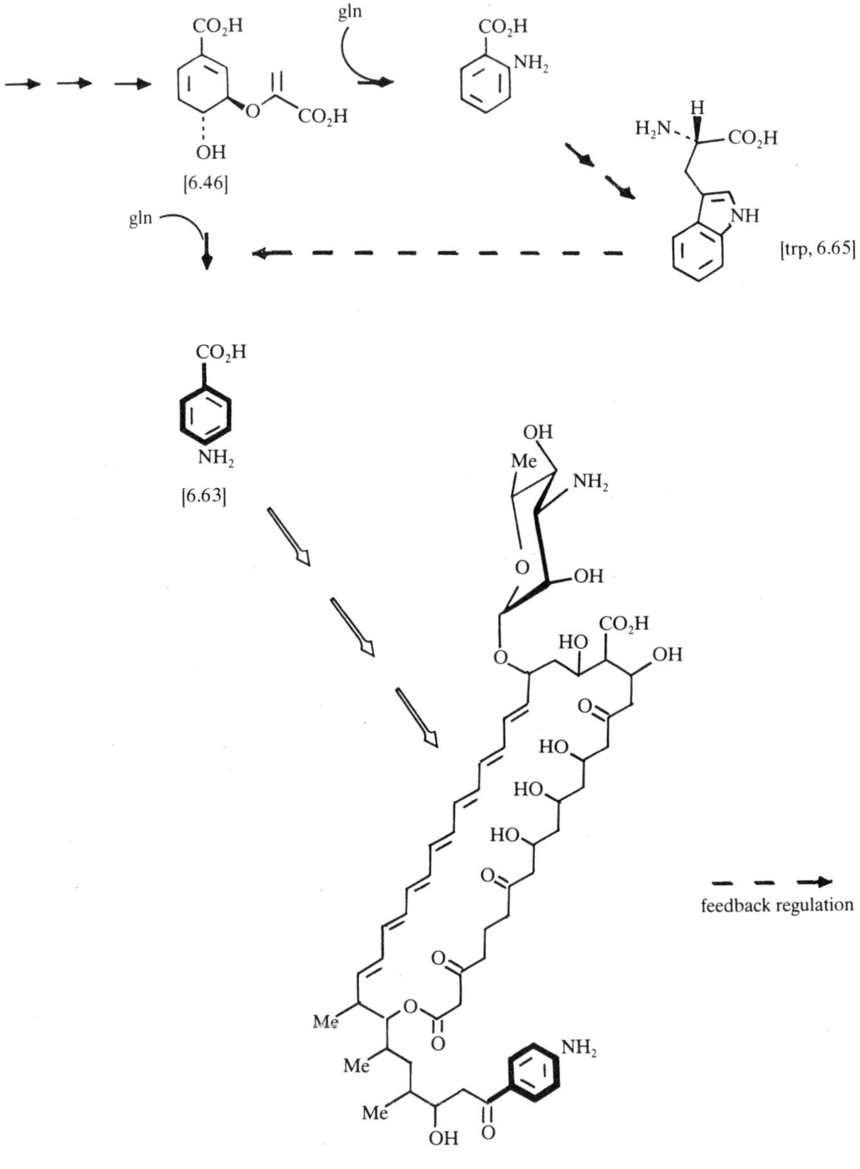

[6.46]

[6.63]

[trp, 6.65]

[candicidin D, 6.64]

feedback regulation

Scheme 6.14. Biosynthesis of candicidin: regulation by L-tryptophan.

References

1. KATZ, E. and DEMAIN, A. L. *Bact. Rev.* **41**, 449 (1977).
BU'LOCK, J. D. *The biosynthesis of natural products*. McGraw-Hill, London (1965).
DEMAIN, A. L. *Lloydia* **31**, 395 (1968).
BU'LOCK, J. D., DETROY, R. W., HOSTALEK, Z., and MUNIM-AL-SHAKARCHI, A. *Trans. Pr. Mycol. Soc.* **62**, 377 (1974).
MARTIN, J. F. and DEMAIN, A. L. *Microbiol. Rev.* **44**, 230 (1980).
BU'LOCK, J. D. in *The biosynthesis of mycotoxins* (ed. P. S. Steyn), p. 1. Academic Press, London and New York (1980).

2. MALIK, V. S. *Adv. appl. microbiol.* **15**, 297 (1972).
VINING, L. C., MALIK, V. S., and WESTLAKE, D. W. S. *Lloydia* **31**, 355 (1968).

3. KRUPINSKY, V. M., ROBBERS, V. E. and FLOSS, H. G. *J. Bact.* **125**, 158 (1976).
FLOSS, H. G. and ANDERSON, J. A. in *The biosynthesis of mycotoxins* (ed. P. S. Steyn), p. 18. Academic Press, London and New York (1980).

4. MOTHES, K. *Secondary plant products*, Vol. 8 (ed. E. A. Bell and B. V. Charlwood), p. 1. Springer-Verlag, Heidelberg and New York (1980).

5. BU'LOCK, J. D. in *The biosynthesis of mycotoxins* (ed. P. S. Steyn), p. 1. Academic Press, London and New York (1980).

6. FOWLER, M. W. *Chem. & Ind.* 229 (1981); *Trans. biochem. Soc.* **11**, 23 (1983).
DOUGALL, K. D. in *Plant cell and tissue culture—principle and application*, p. 727. Ohio State University, Columbus (1979).
DOUGALL, D. K. *The biochemistry of plants*, Vol. 7 (ed. E. E. Conn), p. 21. Academic Press, London and New York (1981).

7. WINK, M., HARTMANN, T., WITTE, I., and SCHIEBEL, H. M. *J. Nat Products* **44**, 14 (1981).

8. HASLAM, E. *Fortschr. Chem. Org. Naturstoffe* **41**, 1 (1982).
GUPTA, R. K., HADDOCK, E. A., and HASLAM, E. *J. Chem. Soc., Perkin Transactions 1* 2535 (1982).

9. BU'LOCK, J. D., DETROY, R. W., HOSTOLEK, Z., and MUNIM-AL-SHAKARCHI, A. *Trans. Br. Mycol. Soc.* **62**, 377 (1974).

10. WOODRUFF, H. B. *Soc. Gen. Microbiol. Symp.* **16**, 22 (1966).
FOSTER, J. W. *Bact. Rev.* **11**, 167 (1947).
WEINBERG, E. D. *Persp. Biol. Med.* **14**, 565 (1971).

11. BRIAN, P. W. *Soc. Gen. Microbiol. Symp.* **7**, 168 (1957).

12. FRAENKEL, G. S. *Science* **129**, 1466 (1959).

13. EHRLICH, P. R. and RAVEN, P. H. *Evolution* **18**, 586 (1965).

14. JANZEN, D. H. *Science* **164**, 415 (1969).

15. MULLER, C. H. *Scinece* **164**, 197 415 (1969).

16. RHOADES, D. F. *Herbivores—their interactions with secondary plant*

metabolites (ed. G. A. Rosenthal and D. H. Janzen), p. 3. Academic Press, London and New York (1979).
JANZEN, D. H. ibid., p. 331.

17. GRISEBACH, H. and EBEL, J. *Angew. Chem. int. edn* **17**, 635 (1978).

18. EBEL, J., AYERS, A. R. and ALBERSHEIM, P. *Pl. Physiol.* **57**, 775 (1976).

19. LEA, P. S. and FOWDEN, L. in *Herbivores—their interactions with secondary plant metabolites* (ed. G. A. Rosenthal and D. H. Janzen), p. 135. Academic Press, London and New York (1979).
DEMAIN, A. L. *Ann. N.Y. Acad. Sci.* **235**, 601 (1974).

20. DEMAIN, A. L. *Adv. appl. Microbiol.* **16**, 177 (1973).

21. HARBORNE, J. B. *Introduction to ecological biochemistry.* Academic Press, London and New York (1977).
MULLER, C. H. and CHOU, C.-H. in *Phytochemical ecology* ed. J. B. Harborne), p. 201. Academic Press, London and New York (1972).

22. BROWN, S. A. in *The biochemistry of plant*, Vol. 7 (ed. E. E. Conn), p. 269. Academic Press, London and New York (1981).

23. NEWMAN, E. I. in *Biochemical aspects of plant and animal coevolution* (ed. J. B. Harborne), p. 327. Academic Press, London and New York (1978).

24. JENSEN, R. A. *A. Rev. Microbiol.* **30**, 409 (1976).

25. BU'LOCK, J. D. in *Comprehensive organic chemistry*, Vol. 5 (ed. E. Haslam), p. 927. Pergamon, Oxford (1979).
QUEENER, S. W., SEBEK, O. K., and VEZINA, C. *A. Rev. Microbiol.* **32**, 593 (1978).

26. VANEK, Z., HOSTOLEK, Z., BLUMAUERORA, M., MIBULIK, M., PODEZIL, M., BEHAL, V., and JECHORA, V. *J. pure & appl. Chem.* **34**, 463 (1973).

27. BALDWIN, J. E., JOHNSON, B. L., USHER, J. J., ABRAHAM, E. P., HUDDLESTON, J. A., and WHITE, R. L. *J. Chem. Soc., Chem. Commun.* 1271 (1980).
BAHADUR, G. A., BALDWIN, J. E., USHER, J. J., ABRAHAM, E. P., JAYATILAKE, G. S., and WHITE, R. L. *J. Am. Chem. Soc.* **103**, 7650 (1981).
BALDWIN, J. E., ABRAHAM, E. P., ADLINGTON, R. M., MURPHY, J. A., GREEN, N. B., TING, H.-H., and USHER, J. J. *J. Chem. Soc. Chem. Comm.* 1319 (1983).

28. KJAER, A. and LARSEN, P. O. *Biosynthesis*, Specialist Periodical Reports, Chemical Society, London, **2**, 171 (1973); **4**, 179 (1975); **6**, 155 (1977).

29. FOWDEN, L. in *Biosynthesis and its control in plants* (ed. B. V. Milborrow), p. 49. Academic Press, London and New York (1973).

30. LARSEN, P. O., ONDERKA, D. K., and FLOSS, H. G. *J. Chem. Soc., Chem. Commun.* 842 (1972); *Biochim. biophys. Acta* **381**, 397 (1975).

31. ROSENTHAL, G. A. *Pl. Physiol.* **50**, 328 (1972); *Q. Rev. Biol.* **52**, 155 (1977).

32. FLOSS, H. G. and ANDERSON, J. A. in *The biosynthesis of mycotoxins*

(ed. P. S. Steyn), p. 18. Academic Press, London and New York (1980).

33. ZAMIR, L. O. in *The biosynthesis of mycotoxins* (ed. P. S. Steyn), p. 223. Academic Press, London and New York (1980).

34. LYNEN, F. *J. pure & appl. Chem.* **14**, 137 (1967). MURPHY, G. and LYNEN, F. *Eur. J. Biochem.* **58**, 467 (1975). SCOTT, A. I., BEADLING, L. C., GEORGOPADAKOU, N. H., and SUBARAYAN, C. R. *Bio-org. Chem.* **3**, 238 (1974).

35. RUEFFER, M., NAGAKURA, N., and ZENK, M. H. *Tetrahedron Lett.* 1593 (1978). STÖCKIGT, J., RUEFFER, M., ZENK, M. H., and HOYER, G. A. *Planta Medica* **33**, 188 (1978).

36. HAHLBROCK, K. in *The biochemistry of plants*, Vol. 7 (ed. E. E. Conn), p. 425. Academic Press, London and New York (1981).

37. MALIK, V. S. and VINING, L. C. *Can. J. Microbiol.* **18**, 137 (1972).

38. MARTIN, J.-F. in *Antibiotics and other secondary metabolites* (ed. R. Hutter, T. Leisinger, J. Nüesch, and W. Wehrli), p. 19. Academic Press, London and New York (1978).

SECONDARY METABOLISM—OVERFLOW METABOLISM AN INTERPRETATION?

'Comment is free, but facts are sacred'
C. P. Scott

Cellular metabolism is a complex network of chemical reactions whose twofold purpose is to release energy and to create new cellular material. The interconversion and breakdown of sugars is of prime importance, not only as an energy-yielding process but also as a source of biosynthetic intermediates.[1] Two pathways are of particular significance—the glycolytic sequence, and the citrate or tricarboxylic acid cycle. Together, these account for the bulk of carbohydrate metabolism in most organisms. An alternative route for the oxidation of carbohydrates—the pentose phosphate pathway—although quantitatively of less importance than the glycolytic pathway and the tricarboxylic acid cycle, is nevertheless essential to the proper functioning of metabolism. Together, these pathways provide the principal starting materials (hexose, pentose, tetrose and triose phosphates, pyruvate and phosphoenolypyruvate, oxaloacetate and α-ketoglutarate, acetyl and succinyl coenzyme A) for the synthesis of cellular materials. However, since these pathways have dual roles, both in the synthesis and breakdown of cellular material, they are frequently referred to as amphibolic sequences.

Metabolic regulation[2] is exerted primarily at the initiation of a biosynthetic sequence, and at branch-points where an intermediate partitions between two or more pathways. At the enzymic level this biosynthetic control may be exercised broadly in two ways (*vide supra*)—by the control of enzyme synthesis, and by regulation of enzyme activity. Regulation of the metabolic flux through amphibolic pathways—such as the glycolytic sequence—must also necessarily reflect the dual purpose which these pathways serve. In principle, they should respond to at least two signals—one which indicates the need of the cell for the products of these pathways, and a signal which reflects the state of the energy resources of the cell. In this particular context, Atkinson[3] has elaborated on the concept of the adenylate charge $\left[\dfrac{\text{ATP} + \frac{1}{2}\text{ADP}}{\text{ATP} + \text{ADP} + \text{AMP}}\right]$ in the cell as an indicator of the cell's need to refurbish its supply of ATP, and as a gross regulator of key enzyme activities. Nevertheless, our understanding of how all these various types of regulatory mechanisms interact and finally integrate at the cellular level remains, at best, fragmentary. In particular, the question as to whether, in the overall strategy of the cell, there is any key or master control point of both catabolic and anabolic metabolism, is still an intriguing one. It is pertinent to note, however, in relation to the ensuing discussion, that Atkinson has proposed that the major branch point between catabolism and anabolism occurs at pyruvate or phosphoenolpyruvate in aerobic heterotrophs.

The channelling of metabolites along a particular metabolic sequence is achieved using enzyme catalysts which promote reactions, the relative rates of which, compared to undesirable non-enzymatic reactions of the same substrate, are extremely high (10^6-10^{14}). This enables the cell to work with metabolite concentrations which are very low. Thus, primary products such as the intermediates of the tricarboxylic cycle, amino-acids, etc., do not normally accumulate to a substantial level in cells. The regulation and co-ordination of cellular activity is, however, frequently not perfect. The formation of industrially important primary products of metabolism (e.g. citric acid[4]—*Aspergillus niger*; L-glutamic acid[4]—*Corynebacterium glutamicum*, riboflavin[5]—*Ashbya gossypii*, etc.) exploits these metabolic inefficiencies, and frequently emphasizes them by growing the micro-organism under conditions that further displace the metabolism from normal. Citric acid accumulates to very high levels, and in terms of gross quantities it is the major commercial product derived from filamentous fungi. Citric-acid formation in *Aspergillus niger* appears to result from the operation of the tricarboxylic acid cycle under conditions (e.g. low pH, deficiency of metallic ion cofactors) in which further transformation of the acid is blocked. The mechanism of this inhibition is not yet known. In contrast, Kornberg[6] has suggested that the glyoxylate cycle may account for the accumulation of fumaric acid [7.1] by certain strains of *Rhizopus nigricans*. Acid production by *Rhizopus nigricans* appears to be the result of a continuation of the normal anaplerotic pathway under conditions where further cellular growth is restricted. The excess C-4 acid metabolized accumulates as fumaric acid.

$$\underset{[7.1]}{\overset{\displaystyle HO_2C \diagdown \quad \diagup H}{\underset{\displaystyle H \diagup \quad \diagdown CO_2H}{\|}}}$$

Likewise, plants can accumulate quantities of what are clearly important primary metabolites. Thus it is appropriate to note that citric acid and L-malic acid are key intermediates in the tricarboxylic acid cycle and are isolable, as Scheele first demonstrated, from various types of fruit. Shikimic acid ([7.2] Scheme 7.1) is a key intermediate[7] in the pathway of aromatic amino-acid metabolism which takes its name. The acid can usually be found in most green plant tissues and in some it occurs in substantial quantities, e.g. star aniseed (Shikimi-no-ki). Alongside shikimic acid [7.2] in plants, the closely-related quinic acid [7.3] is invariably discerned, often in substantially greater amounts than [7.2]. In bacteria, this acid [7.3] has been unequivocally shown *not* to be an obligatory intermediate in the pathway of aromatic amino-acid metabolism. Its frequent occurrence in plants, and its relationship to 3-dehydroquinic acid [7.4], suggests that it is a 'shunt' or 'overflow' metabolite derived from the

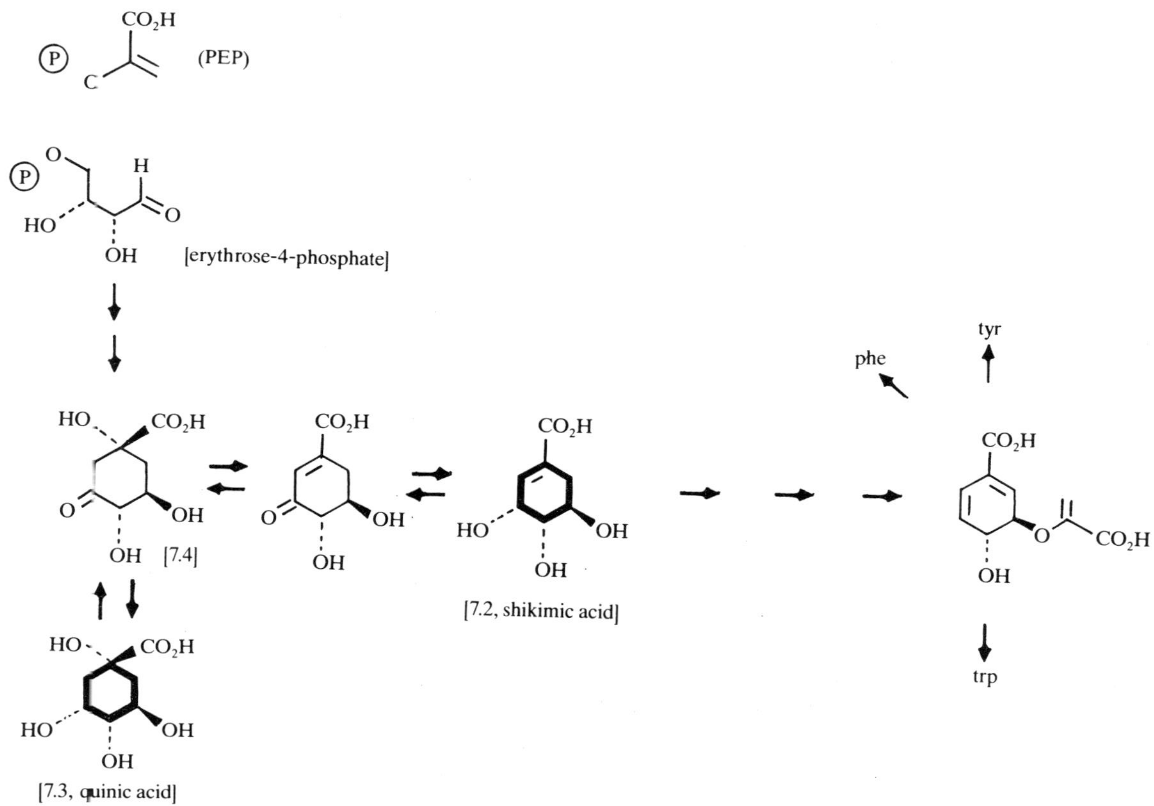

Scheme 7.1. The shikimate pathway in higher plants—an outline.[7]

nomal operation of the pathway by the reduction of [7.4]. By analogy, the accumulation of the primary metabolite shikimic acid [7.2], alongside quinic acid [7.3], points unmistakably to some limiting enzymic process after the intermediate shikimic acid [7.2] in the operation of the shikimate pathway (Scheme 7.1) in higher plants.

In contradistinction, secondary metabolites are regularly found stored in the organism or in its immediate environment, often in large quantities. Leaves of the tea plant (*Cammellia sinensis*), may, for example, store up to 40 per cent of their dry weight as phenolic secondary metabolites. The idea that these substances were 'overflow' or 'shunt' metabolites was first expressed by Foster,[9] and later embroidered, decorated, and developed by other workers. This hypothesis holds that secondary metabolites arise because the normal metabolism of the organism has become unbalanced, and substrate (primary or intermediary metabolite) molecules accumulate—as such, or in a transformed state, often with a complex and unusual structure (secondary metabolite).

The *raison d'etre* of secondary metabolism is a biological problem which requires as yet more detailed analysis. The question of the sequence, timing, and control of the reactions involved in secondary metabolism remains largely unexplained. Of the various ideas put forward, that of 'shunt' or 'overflow' metabolism has, in its various modifications, nevertheless continued to attract attention. In seeking to explore and perhaps provide further evidence in support of this hypothesis, it is interesting to note that a great many secondary metabolites have in common the fact that their biosynthesis originates from just a few key intermediates of primary metabolism (Scheme 7.2)—for example, phosphoenolpyruvate [7.5], pyruvate [7.6], acetyl coenzyme A [7.7], and 3-phosphoglyceric acid [7.8], plus principally (although not exclusively) those protein α-amino-acids synthesized directly from these intermediates, e.g. L-alanine, or by multi-step pathways# from them (Scheme 7.2, e.g. the various aromatic amino-acids). This latter group of α-amino-acids are those for which, in the Atkinson terminology, the metabolic costs are high, and they are formed via biosynthetic sequences discarded by higher organisms during the course of evolution (e.g. L-leucine, isoleucine, valine, phenylalanine, tyrosine, trypto-phan and lysine). The common feature which inter-relates the intermediates [7.5]-[7.8] is that they occur as the final part of the glycolytic sequence and immediately prior to entry into the tricarboxylic acid cycle. These two observa-tions taken together, support the suggestion that secondary metabolism may be related to a change in metabolism of the producer organism from one of normal sustained growth to one in which there is a decreased uptake of acetyl coenzyme A into the tricarboxylic acid cycle, probably reflecting a diminished need in the organism for the supply of nucleotide triphosphates.[3] Whatever the immediate cause of this event (e.g. nutrient depletion and limitation, change in external growth conditions such as pH, etc.), secondary metabolism can, in these terms, be visualized as a means of siphoning away those intermediates directly prior to entry into the tricarboxylic acid cycle (Scheme 7.2). The

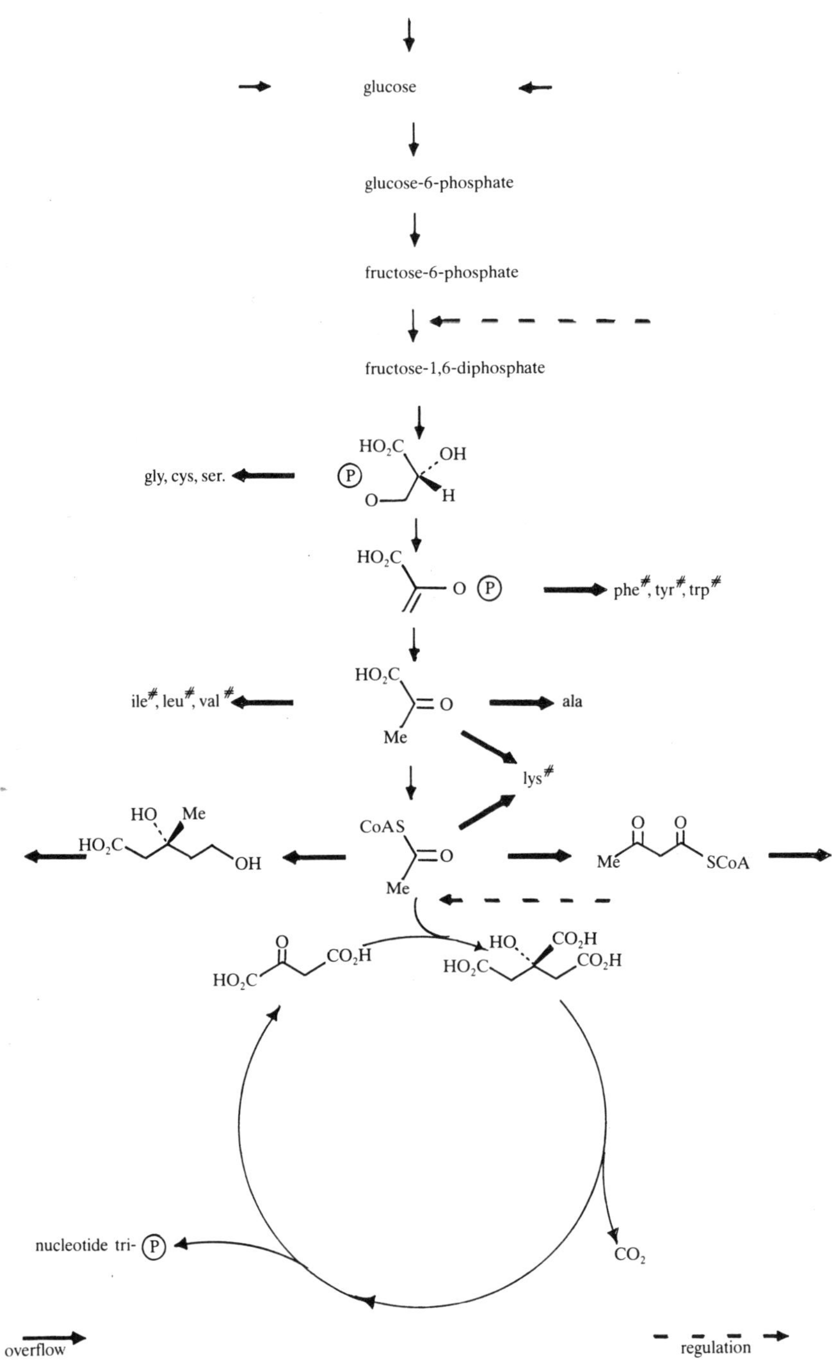

Scheme 7.2. Secondary metabolites—biosynthetic origins. Overflow metabolism?

physiology of metabolite over production, of which secondary metabolism would then be an example, is not a well-understood phenomenon, but it is significant to note that in a study of product formation in various nutrient-limited chemostat cultures of *Klebsiella aerogenes*, Neijssel and Tempest[10] observed that acetate, and often pyruvate, were produced under almost all conditions of growth limitation. Similar experiments with *Escherichia coli* grown in a sulphate-limited chemostat on glucose, produced large quantities of acetate but not pyruvate. The authors interestingly concluded from these observations that under the particular conditions of growth-limitation, the rate of glycolysis in the particular organism was generally exceeding the capacity of the tricarboxylic acid cycle, and was thus producing a build-up of intermediates prior to entry to the cycle. The analogy to the suggested rationale (Scheme 7.2) for secondary metabolism is a clear one. In the experiments of Neijssel and Tempest, the overflow of metabolites before the tricarboxylic acid cycle results in a direct discharge of some of these intermediates (e.g. pyruvate and acetate). In the case of secondary metabolism in plants and micro-organisms, it is possible that these same intermediates, and α-amino-acids derived from them, are then variously transformed by induced secondary processes into a range of secondary metabolites. As Bu'Lock succinctly remarked[11] in 1965, 'secondary metabolism would thus appear to provide organisms with a means of adjustment to changing circumstances'.

References

1. YUDKIN, M. and OFFORD, R. *Comprehensible biochemistry*. Longman, London (1973).
2. LARNER, J. *Intermediary metabolism and its regulation*. Prentice Hall, New York (1971).
3. ATKINSON, D. E. *Cellular energy metabolism and its regulation*. Academic Press, London and New York (1977); *Curr. Topic Cell Regul.* **1**, 29 (1969).
4. MIALL, L. M. in *Economic microbiology*, Vol. 2 (ed. A. H. Rose), p. 47. Academic Press, London and New York (1978).
   KINOSHITA, S. and NAKAYAMA, K., ibid., p. 209.
5. DEMAIN, A. L. *Rev. Microbiol.* **26**, 369 (1972).
6. KORNBERG, H. A. *Rev. Microbiol.* **13**, 49 (1959).
7. HASLAM, E. *The shikimate pathway*. Butterworths, London (1974).
8. HASLAM, E. in *Biochemistry of plant phenolics*, Vol. 12, *Recent advances in phytochemistry* (ed. T. Swain, J. B. Harborne, and C. F. van Sumere), p. 475. Plenum Press, New York (1979).
9. FOSTER, J. W. *Bact. Rev.* **11**, 167 (1947).
10. NEIJSSEL, O. M. and TEMPEST, D. W. *Soc. Gen. Microbiol. Symp.* **29**, 53 (1979).
11. BU'LOCK, J. D. *Biosynthesis of natural products*, p. 11. McGraw-Hill, London (1965).

SPECIES INDEX

SUBJECT INDEX

(Prefixes have been discounted in alphabetizing the entries.)